Mandy,
Thank you so
much for your
support!
xo
Barb.

Go Goddess!

From Depleted to Divine

Barb Thomas, RHN
and Jennifer Rochford

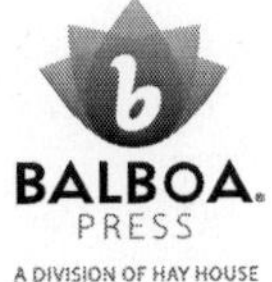

To contact the authors, please email barb@love2eat.ca

Balboa Press books may be ordered through booksellers or by contacting:

Balboa Press
A Division of Hay House
1663 Liberty Drive
Bloomington, IN 47403
www.balboapress.com
1-(877) 407-4847

ISBN: 978-1-4525-3620-0 (sc)
ISBN: 978-1-4525-3619-4 (hc)
ISBN: 978-1-4525-3621-7 (e)

Library of Congress Control Number: 2011911413

Printed in the United States of America

Balboa Press rev. date: 09/23/2011

The authors do not advocate the use of any particular treatment program, but believe that the information presented in this book should be available to the public. The nutritional and health information presented in their book is based on the research, training and personal experiences of the authors, and is true and complete to the best of the authors' knowledge. However, this book is intended only as an informative guide for those wishing to know more about good heath and lifestyle balance. It is not intended to replace or countermand the advice given by the reader's trained health professional. Because there is always some risk involved, the authors are not responsible for any adverse effects or consequences resulting from any of the suggestions made in this book. Because each person and situation is unique, the authors urge the reader to consult with a qualified healthcare professional before using any procedure where there is a question as to its appropriateness.

To every woman who has unconditionally leant their support to us, loved us, and granted us the divine gift of their goddess wisdom.

We are honored to call you sister, mother, daughter, friend.

Thank you.

Contained Within

Introducing The Goddess xi

Part One: Care of the Goddess Temple 1

Chapter One, Nourish 3
Chapter Two, Hydrate 33
Chapter Three, Breathe 39
Chapter Four, Movement 45
Chapter Five, SPA 55

Part Two: Care of the Goddess Spirit 63

Chapter Six, Inspiration 65
Chapter Seven, Spirit 75
Chapter Eight, Get Real Goddess 93

Part Three: The Revolution 97

Chapter Nine, The Revolution 99
Chapter Ten, The Recipes 109

Resources 123
Acknowledgments 125
About the Goddesses 127

Introducing The Goddess

God may be in the details, but the
Goddess is in the questions.
Once we begin to ask them,
there's no turning back.

-Gloria Steinem

Well, Goddess. You have picked up this book. Good for you! We know that right now, as you read this, you probably don't feel very Goddessy. Or you WANT to feel Goddessy, but you are not sure why. Or you just know, deep in your heart, that you should be taking better care of yourself, but you don't know where to start. We have written this book for you.

The Goddess knows that women are important. The Goddess knows that women are vital to the survival of our species and the survival of Mother Earth, too. But most of all, the Goddess knows that there has GOT to be something better than the feelings of exhaustion, of not being good enough, of not being able to keep up with the world that she lives in, every day. There's too much laundry, too much work, not enough time to spend cherishing children, to read a good book, to even just rest- to breathe fresh air - for even a minute.

We've heard your cries. Your body hurts, your mind is tired, and you know that things, on the inside, just aren't working quite right. You are down on yourself. You feel too fat, too skinny, not smart enough, not happy enough, not able to cope. The Goddess inside you knows all this, too, and she is sad. Goddess, you say? Yes, you ARE a Goddess, and from this moment on, we will only refer to you this way. So get used to it... we did.

Oh Goddess, be strong. We, as fellow Goddesses who have been-there-done-that in huge ways, countless times, are here for you. This book is meant to be a love letter to you, the women who have the potential to change their lives and change the world. We want you to feel as good as we do now. We want you to figure things out. As a Holistic Nutritionist and a Spiritual Counsellor, as mothers, as WOMEN, we talk to other gals every day who feel like you do. This book is the culmination of our own bumblings and searchings, of the victories of countless women we have counseled, mentored, and taught. Women who started out just like you.

We also feel it necessary to say something else to you. We know you exist in the Real World. This is the world where deadlines make you stay up until midnight, where, if you are a mother, there are days where you can be peed on, pooped on, spit up on and thrown up on all at the same time. We know that there are real stressors out there that make giving any attention to yourself seem like it is completely a pipe dream. We know sometimes you could go for days without showering if you have a new baby, where 5 a.m. hockey practice means your breakfast dishes don't get done til five p.m. We know this world, and we live it every day too.

When we were both in our early thirties, in the throes of motherhood and wifedom and careerdom, we used to comb through the bookstores, desperately searching for something to help us understand the loss of the sense of self we were both feeling. We would talk about it for hours on the phone together, tossing all kinds of ideas around as to why we couldn't seem to pull ourselves out of the tiredness, the confusion and the fuzziheadedness we were both feeling. We talked about how we knew there must be more to life than what we were currently experiencing, yet every time we looked for some point of reference - some sort of owner's manual about how to function (and succeed!) in spades - at being a woman, we always fell short. We promised each other we would figure it out, and we have. We are now sharing what we have learned with you.

We have written this book to be like a road map for you, but we have written in from a place and a time in our lives where things like spit up, dishes and laundry are still very real for us. We have made changes. And these changes have enriched our lives in unimaginable ways.

Our commitment to you is that as you read this, you will feel assured that the changes we are suggesting YOU can make work in very practical ways, in a very raw and real world.

Here's how this book works. Each chapter contains three sections:

- "Get Ready" introduces you to the concept of the chapter.
- "Get Set" gives you the tools you need to feel confident enough to make a change.
- "Go Goddess!" asks you to try one simple thing that you can incorporate quickly into your busy days, but which can have a profound effect on the *quality* of your life.

We invite you to first read the book cover to cover, but once you get the gist of it, feel free to use it more as a reference book, accessing the sections you need when you are feeling low, or like you need a boost, or to come back on centre. It's kind of like a life preserver. Toss a chapter or two to yourself when you need to stay afloat. Eventually, all the things we recommend will become like breathing. You will just know to do it, without having to think about it.

Goddess, it's time to begin your journey. And don't worry, it's not scary, and it's not overwhelming. We will see to that. Your journey begins here, with just the simple turn of a page, and ends... well hopefully it never does. But there is one thing we know for sure. We are ready to help you travel, and keep you gliding down a road that is light, that is vibrant, that is joyful, that is revolutionary. Just like you....

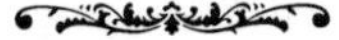

Goddessing without Guilt

Guilt. Ugh. What an ugly word. Who needs it? Certainly not the Goddesses! Well, good news. This book is guilt free!

Many women feel that guilt needs to be attached to caring for themselves or putting themselves first. We will go deeper into this concept later in the book, but for now, you need only to be clear about the important, self "ful" reasons to make Goddessy choices. Often, when we see a woman making self "ish" choices, we refer to her as a Diva. Think of the movie starlet who would only accept white lilies in her dressing room.

There is a HUGE difference between being a self serving Diva, and living out loud as a Goddess. So you can continue to read this book GUILT FREE, we have included a handy chart to help set you straight.

Diva	Goddess
Believes there is nothing more important than her own pleasure.	Knows that her own internal joyfulness comes first, so she can be a woman strong enough to help heal the Earth.
Believes having power over others makes her better than others.	Knows that with internal strength, she can be a powerful role model for other humans.
Demands	Manifests
Is selfISH	Is self-FULL
Is controlled by EGO.	Lives in the present, in Joy, where EGO does not live.

Got it? GREAT! Let's Go Goddess!

Part One:
Care of the Goddess Temple

CHAPTER ONE

Nourish

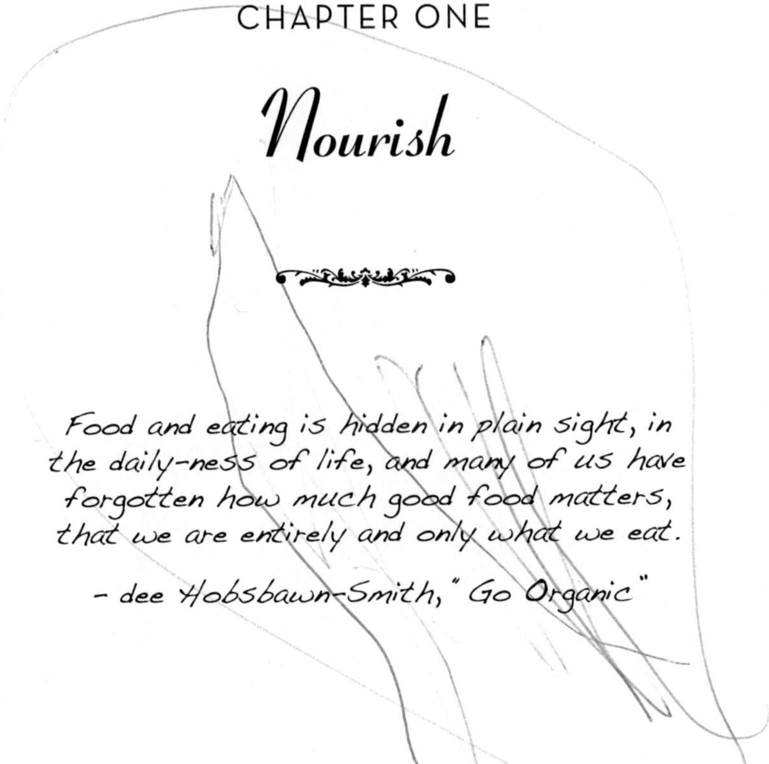

Food and eating is hidden in plain sight, in the daily-ness of life, and many of us have forgotten how much good food matters, that we are entirely and only what we eat.

– dee Hobsbawn-Smith, "Go Organic"

Nourish

Get Ready...

The care and feeding of the Goddess starts deep within. There is no simpler way to say it: until you begin to foster the deep, undying respect that you so deserve for yourself, you will never see significant change physically or spiritually. Years of self abuse and neglect can make self respect a hard commodity to come by. But it needn't be earned. You already have it, far down inside you. It is astounding how awfully we, as women, treat ourselves! We continuously put our needs last, we push ourselves a little too hard, we call ourselves degrading names like fat, ugly, stupid. Is this how we would treat our best friend? Of course not. What kind of respectful friend would we be if we did? Before we discuss with you what will best carry your physical form forward - what will nourish you on the most basic level, we feel it necessary to discuss the biggest question of all in relation to nourishment - why do we eat?

Emotional Eating

The term "Emotional Eating" is such a buzz word right now in the media. It is a term used to describe how we use food to abuse our bodies and cope with our lives, much the same as the way a drug addict would use heroin. Modern pop psychology has led us to believe that food should only be used as fuel, and that if we use it for comfort or coping we are weak, and abusing it and ourselves.

We have counseled so many women who have sat and cried in our sessions over the guilt they feel when they abuse food. It is so heartbreaking to see how these women have such a low opinion of themselves, and how their own identities are drowning in the regret they feel about their food and coping choices.

Goddess has her own opinion about emotions and food.

We, as women and Goddesses, are innately emotional creatures. This is something we should neither try to hide nor feel shame about. Every action we take in life has an emotional connection behind it. When we apply this to the subject of nourishment, it is not hard to understand that every choice we make, from shopping and selecting food, to preparing it for ourselves and our families, to actually eating it, is done with emotion.

When we shop for our families, we are selecting the food we will give them with love and concern for their health. When we prepare meals for our friends and loved ones, we feel pride when they tell us that it was delicious and that they are satisfied. When we eat it ourselves, however, we often choose feelings such as guilt and remorse in relation to our actions. And this is where emotional eating comes into play.

The more we make choices that make us feel guilty, the worse we feel, and the more we eat. The more we eat, the more respect we lose for ourselves, and so the cycle continues. How is it that we are able to lovingly take the time to select the best foods for the people we care about, take the time to craft beautiful dishes that come from our heart, and then, when we sit down to take part in the meal ourselves, we are wracked with guilt?

Emotional eating does not have to be a negative thing! When you internalize the idea that you are so significant to the existence of this, the human race, then you will be able to experience the love and respect that you rightfully deserve, yet often deny yourself. We are here to tell you that it is perfectly fine to be an emotional eater. Just choose the right emotion! Put passion and love into every experience surrounding food. Turn your shopping trips and cooking experiences into ways of showing love to yourself, not just your family. Choose the best quality food that you can afford, prepare each dish, even a simple sandwich, with love and awe for your body and spirit and then, when you sit down to consume what you have crafted, make the choice to eat it, regardless of what it is, from a place of joy! Choose **joy** as your primary emotion surrounding food. Remember, when you are able to stand in awe and regard your body with the respect it deserves, then you will only want to make joyful choices for it.

Of course we understand that there are many layers for some in regards to their food addictions and struggles. However, we also know that they all stem from the same place - a place and a time, long ago, when the consciousness of the planet, held in our cells still to this very day, made women feel insignificant and worthless.

We still feel it, even though things are a little better for us, here on Earth. It is time, right now, Goddess, to kick that social paradigm out on its butt. It's time for you to know, on the deepest level, that YOU - who you are right this moment - are absolutely perfect in every way. Perfect for this, the journey that you are meant to be on. This is not to say that you don't have a lot of learning and growing to do, but in this moment, right now, the miracle of your body and soul stands naked, waiting for you to acknowledge it. So 300 pounds or 80 pounds, you need to right now stop creating your identity around your negative choices and behaviors, and start loving the wisdom of your body and soul, as it has chosen to cope in the best way that it knows how. Forgive yourself for any time you feel you have wronged yourself. That is in the past, and you don't live there. You live here, in the present, where everything is as it should be. Every moment is an opportunity to make new choices that will enrich your life. KNOW that you are powerful. KNOW that you are worth every ounce of respect you can muster, and don't let anyone tell you any different. When a nice, juicy layer of respect sits simmering at the foundation of your spirit, then making your food choices from a place of joy begins to seem so very logical.

Now that you know the *why*, let's talk about the *what* and *how*. If you are ready to make these amazing and simple choices for your body and soul, then you are going to need a little road map, and we will even throw in an anatomy lesson for you. We believe that the more you know about the awesome function of your body, the more power you will have to make joyful choices. So follow along, and see if any of the next part of the book resonates for you, and helps direct you to making more graceful choices for your beautiful self.

Mindful Eating, Guilt Free

Let's say you're at your in-laws' house for a holiday meal, and there, on the table lies a plate of Aunt Helga's decadent, mouthwatering, homemade brownies. My, but do they look good. And here's the thing. You have already had dinner. Uh oh. Here comes the eternal conundrum: Do you reach for a brownie? Here's how you decide....

The Brownie Exercise- Finding the Joy

First, ask yourself your question: "Can I make this choice from a place of joy? Can I eat this brownie with no guilt, no shame, knowing that it may not be the best choice for my waistline, but sure as heck may satisfy my soul? Can I?" If the answer is yes, then guess what? It's time to eat the brownie. Crazy, we know. But here's the thing. There are so many pleasures in life. As a nutritionist, this Goddess will be the first to tell you that refined sugar and white flour are not the best for your body... but on a soul level, nourishment can come in many forms...

Second, practice this regularly (and you don't need to eat a brownie every time). Choose something simple, something good for you, or not, but certainly something that you love to eat, like a strawberry, or a piece of silky dark chocolate. Before you pop it in your mouth, take a moment and hold it in your hands. Send a message of gratitude out to the Universe. Look at what you've selected. Admire its color, its texture. Then hold it up to your nose. Inhale its scent. Then go ahead and pop it in your mouth. Hold it there for a moment and really taste it. Chew slowly, appreciating the textures and flavours that are released. Taste it as if you are tasting it for the first time. Really experience it. Close your eyes and appreciate all the intricacies of the flavor of the food, as you would a fine wine, or as Dr. Christiane Northrup[1] says "as if you were dancing in the moonlight with a lover". Then, after another moment, go ahead and swallow it. Allow yourself a moment to let the taste linger in your mouth, and settle in your body, before you get on with your day.

If you respect your body enough, you will realize that one brownie is not going to tip the scales. One brownie may even bring you joy. If you respect yourself enough, you will know that the next brownie, or maybe the third, would be doing your body a disservice, and you will not chow down. You will not measure your self worth against what you consume, you will not beat yourself up or punish yourself for your choice.

1 Northrup, Christiane, The Power Of Joy (audio recording) Listen to Dr. Northrup's amazing audio recording, The Power of Joy on your mp3 player on the way to work to help stay focussed and joyful!

Willpower

Let's talk about willpower for a second. Willpower indicates that you have some sort of POWER over your mind's own ability to make a choice. Willpower indicates that you are so distrustful of your ability to judge what will serve you and what won't that you have to CONTROL, in a regimented way, the choices that you make, all the while DEPRIVING yourself of things that may bring you joy on some level. How about respect? As women, it is so imperative that we understand how important it is to respect ourselves on a deep, deep level. We must understand deeply that our ability to know what is right for ourselves is always there. It is just usually being ignored. Innately, whether you know it or not, your intuition - your body-mind connection, your GODDESS WISDOM - knows just how much of something you can handle, before it becomes destructive to your body.

Charles Eisenstein, in his book *The Yoga of Eating*[2], says, "Like a young child, your body loves you totally and instinctively. Like a faithful dog, it stays loyal even when you kick and abuse it. What is the proper way to treat a trusting young child? With patience and unconditional love. And that is also the proper way to treat your body."

Care of the Body

The point of this section of the book is to help you to begin to remember how vital self respect and self love are to your survival, the survival of the Goddess, the survival of the feminine. Beginning to care for yourself properly, in the way you deserve, can be very simple. Let's start with our outermost layer, and work inwards. Let's start with the body.

The body is our vehicle that carries us towards enlightenment and true transformation. It deserves our utmost reverence. However, just like a

2 Charles Eisenstein, The Yoga of Eating Washington, New Trends Publishing Inc. 2003 You can learn about the author at www.ascentofhumanity.com

car, if you forget to change your oil, schedule regular maintenance, give it fuel or even take it to the car wash, your vehicle will break down and not be able to take you where you need to go. This is the same for our physical selves. So many women - mothers, career women, students - are moving at such a fast pace and are so busy taking care of others that they forget the first rule of Goddessdom: we must always take care of our vehicle!! Without proper fuel and a smooth running transmission, we inevitably become exhausted over time. Now, we may not notice this at first, this gradual wearing down of our bodies. But let us paint the picture and you can see if it sounds familiar. In the following few paragraphs, we have chosen to use the example of a woman who is a mother. If you are not a mom, hopefully you can still see some of your own life, or your future, reflected in the very typical experience that follows.

Maybe you stayed up late one night catching up on some work. When your alarm goes off at 6:30 a.m., which would leave you enough time to get your morning routine done, you punch the snooze and try to get ten extra minutes. When you finally drag yourself out of bed, you stumble to the coffee pot and immediately turn it on - you need a boost! The kids need to have their lunches made and the dog needs to be fed. Your oldest daughter can't find any socks, so you spend ten minutes rooting through a pile of clean but unfolded laundry on your bedroom floor that you did not have time to put away last night. By this time, you have fifteen minutes to get out the door and you haven't even had a shower. You wash up hastily and grab your makeup to put on in the car. You pour your coffee into a travel mug, help the kids with their backpacks and you all run out the door.

On the way to work there is, of course, a traffic jam putting you another fifteen minutes behind. Well, at least you can put your makeup on while sitting in gridlock. You finally arrive at work, late for a meeting. You run to the meeting and don't get finished until ten. It suddenly hits you that you haven't eaten all morning. Your hands are shaking from all the coffee and your stomach is really starting to hurt. You have to put something in it now! You stagger to the coffee shop down the street and grab, at best, a bagel and cream cheese. Phew. Your day continues this way - squeezing meals in only when it is convenient on the run from meeting to meeting, a granola bar while driving to pick up the kids. At 4:00 p.m., upon returning home, you begin to prepare dinner, but are so hungry by this point that you wolf down half a bag of nacho chips. You quickly make (or heat up) and eat dinner, take the kids to their lessons, help them with their homework and bed time routine, and sit down at 8:00 to fold laundry. You squeeze in an hour of television, at which time you munch on some popcorn, then finish the report you need done for tomorrow. Suddenly it's midnight. You stumble to bed, and hope tomorrow will be a little easier. It isn't. And neither is the next day.

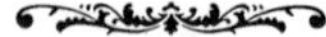

Get Set...

Eating For Energy

On a cellular level, days like the ones we just gave an example of cause great wear and tear. By not providing our bodies with what they truly need, day in and day out, our transmission begins to wear down. Eventually a deep seated exhaustion begins to set in. It becomes harder and harder to go through the grueling pace of our days. Emotionally we begin to wear out as well, because on a physical level we simply do not have the energy we need to do what we feel we need to. We become harder and harder on ourselves and push our bodies and our minds more and more to meet the ridiculous goals we have set for ourselves. We begin to rely on artificial stimulants like caffeine and mood enhancers like antidepressants to help us get through the day. Being a Supercreature - all things to all people - is not only exhausting, it is not truly achievable.

If you could look inside your body and watch it as it went through your busy day, this is what you would see:

To begin: from your first sip of coffee, your adrenal glands, which sit atop your kidneys and are responsible for helping you deal with stress, would begin secreting adrenaline. This would make your heart beat faster. As you move quickly through your morning paces, feeling the mental stress of being late for your day, your body secretes more adrenaline to help you cope. You see, your body does not know the difference between the stress of Primordial You being chased by a tiger, and Modern You, late for work. Since it thinks your stress equals trying to avoid being lunch for a Sabertooth, it faithfully continues to pump out the chemicals that will make you run faster as it tries to save your life.

So, in order to assist you in your escape flight from the tiger, your body in its infinite wisdom shunts blood away from your digestive system and to your limbs, to help you run away from danger. This is all well and fine if you were, in fact, being pursued by a wild animal. But since you are actually standing in your kitchen, wolfing back a bowl of Krunchy Puffs, this is not a good thing! Your stomach and bowels need that blood to do their very important job of helping you digest your food, assimilate your nutrients and ultimately excrete toxic waste.

The health of your entire body depends on these three crucial steps- digestion, absorption and elimination. If there is any sort of block in this chain of command, your health will be sub par at best, and ultimately become a breeding ground for toxins that suck your energy, rob your nutrients and leave you a mess. So how do we ensure our digestive system is functioning optimally? Here is some very useful information, and some handy tips:

Digestion

Digestive issues stem from a variety of places. The Standard American Diet (S.A.D.),which usually consists of foods that are fried, refined, cooked beyond recognition, doused in salt and sugar, and topped of with alcohol and cigarettes, contributes very little to the health of our colon and GI tract. This S.A.D. way of eating is low in fibre, low in water and nutrient deficient, and is how most people in North America eat. To top it off, the day to day amounts of antibiotics and sugar (high fructose corn syrup, glucose-fructose) and other toxins that North Americans intake contribute to the proliferation of bad bacteria (yeast) in the gut. When the balance of your intestinal flora is upset, (the good bugs losing and the bad bugs winning) dysbiosis (the altered balance of intestinal microflora) occurs, and digestion, absorption and elimination are compromised. This generally causes a host of problems within the body from gas and bloating, to skin problems, to a compromised immune system and inflammation. There is nothing more important than a healthy gut!!

Enhancing your digestion then, Goddess, is the necessary first step to more energy and healing.

Important Points on Digestion

- Chew your food to liquid - this requires you to SLOW DOWN!!! (Something we all need to do more of. Your adrenal glands will thank you!)
- Eat mindfully. Eat in a quiet place, with no television or other chaotic distraction, and take the time to taste, smell, and be grateful for your food. This process signals to your body that all is well, there is no tiger chasing you, and no need for extra adrenaline. This way of eating therefore enhances not only your digestion, but how you absorb your nutrients as well. At the end of the meal, allow your body a few minutes to digest before you get up and walk away from the table.
- Eat small meals more often. This takes less energy for your body to digest and provides you with a steady level of blood sugar, which in turn will ensure your energy is regulated throughout the day.

- Have your biggest meal mid-day, as your digestive juices are at their peak at that time, and food digests easier then.

- If you are really having trouble digesting, try eating your proteins (meats, fish, beans) away from your carbohydrates (grains). Proteins and carbs are digested in two different places in your body, so if you eat a sandwich with turkey, for example, or a burger, your body has to use up your precious energy just to first separate the two and send them where they need to go to be digested. This practice of separating your proteins from carbohydrates is called "food combining" and there are many books on the subject. [3]

- Eat fruit on its own, so it does not sit on top of all the other food in your stomach, rotting away (fruit has sugar, which ferments easily). The fermentation process causes gas and bloating and feeds the Yeasty Beasties (bad bacteria) which live in your intestines.

- Do not drink with your meals, as liquid extinguishes the action of your digestive juices. If you are chewing your food to liquid, you should not have to drink to get the food down!

Absorption

Being able to absorb your nutrients is the secret to this whole process. You could eat all the best foods and never miss a day and still be deficient in nutrients. How? If your intestines are bogged down with bad bacteria and toxins, they will be sluggish, and not able to do the job of absorption. All those great nutrients that you thought you were putting

3 Consult with a Nutritionist to see if food combining is right for you.

into your system will just pass right out into the toilet! All three processes are related. If you cannot break your food down (digestion) you won't be able to absorb it. If you are constipated or not able to excrete your waste, it backs up in your system, produces more toxins, feeds the bad bacteria and you then won't be able to absorb new nutrients coming in. Working on enhancing the way your system works from the front to the back door is the best way to do this.

Elimination

So as we said, you need to be sure that for a healthy life, you are able to properly digest your food, absorb your nutrients and excrete what's left over. The topic of excretion is never the most fun, so we will keep it brief. You know in your gut (literally) if your bowels work right.

Bowel function seems to be a hot topic these days, even on tv. Without properly being able to get rid of what you don't need, your energy levels plummet. As well, if waste sits in your bowel for too long, you open yourself up to more dysfunction, more disease, more health issues. Not being able to properly eliminate can be tied to not being able to let go of things you do not need emotionally, as well. Talk to your friendly neighborhood Nutritionist or Naturopathic Doctor if you just can't seem to get a good balance this way, or refer to the book *Eating Alive* by John Matsen, or Dr. Bernard Jensen's *Guide to Better Bowel Care: A Complete Program for Tissue Cleansing Through Bowel Management.*

Absorb the Joy

Here, Goddess, is a list of some of the best foods to nourish you. As you are reading this, remember one thing and you will be nourished, body, mind AND sprit: make all your choices, food choices included, from a place of JOY, every time, without fail. Practice that Brownie Exercise!!

Foods to Favor

For your Grains:

Spelt, quinoa, kamut, rice or flourless, sprouted breads instead of white or even whole wheat. These grains contain less gluten. Less gluten equals less bubbly tummies!

Vegetables:

At least 60% of your diet should be **raw organic vegetables**. This equals about 10-20 half cup (the size of your palm) servings a day. Favour the dark greens like spinach, kale, Swiss chard, collard greens, add in wherever you can. Dark greens can be chopped and tossed on salads or in a soup or stew right before you serve it. Enjoy liberally! Don't forget to use your herbs and fresh oils to kick up the flavour of salads instead of a greasy, preservative laden dressing.

Lemon:

Disease likes to live in an acidic environment. Lemons are extremely detoxifying, alkalizing fruits, even though they taste acidic. Having a glass of lemon water first thing in the morning will help alkalize your system, with the added benefits of kicking your digestive juices into gear, and getting rid of toxins. Drink your lemon water, wait about ten minutes and then check to see if you feel hungry. If you do, this is your body's way of telling you the digestive juices are flowing and your stomach is ready to accept food.

Wild, organic fish:

Especially Wild Alaskan salmon. Salmon contains the much talked about Omega 3 series of Essential Fatty Acids - the good fats that help grow your brain, make your immune system and stop inflammation in its tracks. Fish three times a week would be optimal, but if you can't do it, then make sure you are getting an Omega 3 Fish oil supplement of at least 1000 mg per day.

Coconut Oil:

Oh goodness, how extra virgin, cold pressed, organic coconut oil loves the Goddess, and vice versa! There are so many reasons to love this highly stable oil! First, it has the highest flash point of all oils and therefore will not turn rancid when cooked at high heats. Secondly, coconut oil contains Caprylic Acid which is an anti fungal, and kills the yeastie beasties that inhabit your intestines. Third: it is the Malaysian secret to amazingly healthy skin and hair! We could go on, but for now, just trust us, buy some, and use small amounts of it to start- in baking, on toast, in a stir fry. A word of caution: coconut oil contains magnesium which can loosen your bowels if you dive right in and use a lot in a day. Go easy!

Antioxidant Rich Foods:

These are the foods that prevent your cells from essentially rusting, causing damage and disease. Look for foods that have the highest amounts of antioxidants such as goji berries, blueberries, red and orange peppers, and pomegranate.

Goddess, there are so many wonderful nutrients in our foods, but alas, we will stop here. Nourishment is an amazing subject- we suggest you make it a hobby and learn what you can about the phenomenal foods mother nature provides us. Do you know how to use hemp? Agave syrup? Cacao? Check the back of the book out for more resources, and start a new hobby: whole foods nutrition!!

Go Local

Eating beautiful, nutrient dense food that comes from the Earth not only increases your energy, but allows you to establish a deeper connection with our Mother Earth.

It is profoundly easy in our society for us to lose that connection. We order fast food, we buy meals in shiny boxes from the Big Box Stores and never question where our foods come from. Do we ever stop to ask where our food was grown, how it was handled, what kind of soil it was grown in? Every farmer has a story, and every story needs to be told. Our farmers are the only connection we have to our food these days, unless we grow it ourselves.

The greatest treasure our modern cities hold are the Farmers' Markets that provide us with local, seasonal fare that is so much higher in nutrients than the stuff that sits on trains, trucks, and in the backs of warehouses before it makes it out to the shelves in grocery stores. Part of developing the deep respect for your body that you so deserve is to remember that you deserve the best of everything. Making a conscious decision to buy your food from local growers not only injects money into your local economy and supports the environment, but it also ensures that you are getting the most nutrient dense food out there. A genetically modified watermelon that has come all the way from Peru and has taken a month to get to your plate has far less nutrients than a tomato that was picked yesterday and brought to you by Joe Farmer who lives less than a day away from your house.

The Energy of Food- Quiet vs. Noisy

Begin to pay attention to the ENERGY of food. Can you feel the difference in your body when you eat a locally grown meal that is prepared with love, versus a fast food burger prepared commercially?

When your food is ENERGETIC, your body absorbs it better, and gives that energy to you. This is called quiet food - food that your body knows what to do with, every time you eat it. Quiet food is freshly picked, clean and nutritious. Quiet food is free from artificial colors, flavours, preservatives and things like MSG or human growth hormones and antibiotics. When your body eats quiet food, it knows exactly what to do with the nutrients coming in, and it efficiently sends the nutrients to where they need to go in the body.

On the other hand, when you eat food that contains things like pesticides, hydrogenated oils or trans fats, waxes, dyes, and preservatives, your ever faithful body has to work harder to get rid of them. This is called noisy food - food that creates a back up in your system as your body tries to figure out where to put the things it doesn't recognize. As well, when you eat food that is void of nutrients - products that are refined and processed - your body works to try to balance your system. When your body can't find any minerals from the white sugar you have just eaten, it will balance this lack of nutrients by pulling minerals from your own bones. Noisy food is not just an indulgence, it can be dangerous.

Good, Better, Best

Again though, Goddess, life is about balance, and a beautiful piece of chocolate cake or even a few strips of licorice now and then is not going to be the end of you. The idea is to make the right choice, as often as you can, and for the times you don't, leave them behind and try again to give yourself the gift of good food. You can always count on living by the Goddessy Principle of "Good, Better, Best". "Best", in relation to your food choices, means choosing the kind of quiet food we have listed above, that is clean and nutrient dense, and fuels your body with energy. "Better" would mean choosing food that you know may not be perfect, but still offers you more benefit than something that is processed and refined. For instance, choosing whole grains over white bread. "Good" means, regardless of what opportunity you have, you try to choose at least the best QUALITY of food. For example, if you find yourself making the choice to go to a fast food restaurant, choose the best food that you can while you are there, and eat it without guilt, and with joy. Then, for your next food choice, try to choose something else that better serves you physically.

So be mindful, choose wisely and raise your food consciousness. Connect with the people that matter to food, and you will connect with the food that truly makes a difference to your life.

Goddessy Whole Foods Principles to Live By

- Eat Local Food
- Eat organic whenever you can afford to. Reduce your exposure, and nature's exposure, to toxic chemicals!
- Eat seasonally. Trust that, for the most part, Mother Nature provides us with what we need throughout the year, right in our own back yards.
- Eat as close to the Earth as you can. If it comes in a shiny box, and has words you can't identify, it probably is not doing you any good, and could do you harm. As Michael Pollan, in his excellent, simple to read book, *Food Rules, An Eater's Manual* says, "Avoid food products containing ingredients that no normal human would keep in their pantry."[4] Basically, if you can't recognize the ingredient, your body can't either. Trust in the power of real food.
- Eat clean- avoid additives, preservatives, colours, artificial flavours and trans fats.

4 Pollan, Michael, Food Rules New York, Penguin Books, 2009

- Prepare your foods with joy and love. Take time while you cook to smell your food, sample tastes, feel the textures in your hands and mouth. Make your meal prep time a sensual, decadent experience. VERY Goddessy.

Love that Liver

Be kind to your poor liver! Your liver is responsible for over 500 jobs that we know of. It is such an amazing organ and deserves Goddess reverence. Your liver's number one job, though, is detoxification. If you continually overload your body with things that your liver then has to clean up in order to keep you safe, (things like alcohol, drugs, cigarette smoke, preservatives, and pesticides) your poor liver will be so busy trying to keep you safe from the poisons that it won't be able to properly do some of its other vital jobs, like making a proper balance of hormones. Even your personal care products, such as your shampoos and make-up, and your household cleaners like laundry detergent and floor cleaners contain poisons that your liver has to clean up. For a really excellent, very Goddessy guide to cleaning up your beauty regimen and home in a fun, environmentally conscious way, please read Sophie Uliano's book, *Gorgeously Green*. Raising your Goddess Consciousness in regards to how we are polluting our bodies and Mother Earth is a very Goddessy thing to do.

Take time every day to drink green tea and teas that contain milk thistle or dandelion root to help keep your liver healthy and happy! Indulge in foods that support your liver like lemon, beets, artichokes, garlic and onions. See the recipe section for some fabulous, simple recipes that love your liver!

Be Kind to Your Cortisol

So ok, now you know about your digestive system. Lucky you! But there is another body process that you need to understand if you want to live vitally and full of life. This process, which begins with the adrenal glands, as mentioned earlier, also deals with a hormone called cortisol. Cortisol is the hormone that your hard working adrenal glands make that helps you cope with stress. When you live a life that makes your body think that a tiger is continually chasing you, your adrenal glands become exhausted. They keep up as long as they can, but eventually, they will slow, and sometimes shut down. When the adrenals give up, they produce very little cortisol, and therefore your physiological mechanism to actually handle any kind of stress disappears. You may begin to feel pain in weird places, you may feel depressed, hopeless, sad, fat, and more than anything, really, really tired.

How are we supposed live life to the fullest, be role models for our children, heal ourselves and ultimately heal the planet if we can't even lift our heads off the pillow? Coming back from adrenal fatigue and exhaustion can be a very long road. If you really truly believe you have already hit rock bottom, it is best that you have a good friend help you go about gathering a team of health professionals that can become your safety net and slowly guide you back to health. If you are someone who is not there yet, but feels you are on the road, follow the tips below to help bring yourself back to a place where you can stand in your own power, full of the life and energy that you so very much deserve.

Nutrients for Healthy Adrenals

Foods that contain B vitamins are wonderful for your adrenals. Chop dark green leafy vegetables like spinach, kale, and Swiss Chard very fine and just toss them on your salad. B vitamins are the things that make your body's energy spark plugs go. Also, whole grains like quinoa, oats, barley, buckwheat and spelt are also great for supplying B vitamins. Check out the recipes in the back of this book for great ways to get more B vitamins.

Vitamin C is also extremely supportive for the adrenals. Add berries to your smoothies, and red peppers to your salads. Get friendly with amazing superfoods like goji berries or rooibos tea. Not only will vitamin C help keep your adrenals strong, it will help boost your immunity as well. We have great vitamin C filled recipes in our Recipe section.

Anti-nutrients to Avoid

Any substance that causes your adrenals to work harder will deplete your energy and exhaust you over time. Even though they may give your bursts of energy in the short term, please try to avoid things like refined (white) sugars, caffeine, drugs (including nicotine) and alcohol. Obviously a glass of wine there or a lovely latte here will not damage most people beyond repair, but if you are really trying your best to recover your strength and inject boundless energy and joy into your life, then just be very mindful of how these things make you feel long term. Make the best choice, as always, that is right for you and only you.

Rest and Rejuvenation

The best nutrients for your adrenal glands!

If you are feeling exhausted, you must, must, must rest, dear Goddess. Now is the time for you to really begin to realize the importance of putting yourself first. Cut back on what you are doing in general. If your adrenals need supporting, then it is really important you start saying no to things and dropping what you absolutely don't need to do. We have been there - a couple of babies, or a full time career (or both!) and adrenal exhaustion are a bad mix, and it could take you years to bounce back if you are not proactive. NOW is the time to nip this in the bud. Here are some musts for your NEW, YOU focussed to-do list:

- Pare everything back. Set up a very basic routine for you (and the kids, if you have them). Don't worry about having the house perfect or even tidy at this point. Rest at every opportunity. The laundry will wait!
- Ask for help. Explain to your loved ones, or your partner, what is going on and that you need extra help. Hire cleaning help if you can. If you are a mom, get a good babysitter and actually schedule YOU time into your week during the day. Even one hour a week to just go to a great book store and read by yourself is helpful. Join a moms' group or a book club - even if you don't think it's your thing. It really helps to talk to other women when you feel this way.
- Slow yourself down in the way you accomplish your everyday tasks. The bottom line is, you need to stop the adrenaline from pumping unnecessarily. Chew slower, breathe slower, drive slower, walk slower, talk slower and just BE slower. Slow down before the Universe slows you down with illness or disease.
- Establish a good bedtime routine that is for you. Use the evening to rejuvenate, no matter what your circumstances are. Run a bath with lavender, do a little yoga, read a really good book, meditate and breathe (more on this later!).
- Take every day, minute by minute. Remember, you live HERE, in the present moment. And in the present, everything is perfect. It's the past and the future that

cause anxiety, and that is not where you are, nor can you ever be. You can't worry your way out of a problem, and you need to solve your problems with a higher vibration, or a clearer, calmer mind, than the one that made the problems in the first place. Live for the now, and refuse to accept anything less for yourself. Put yourself first, always. It makes you a better mommy, a better wife, a better woman, a better human. Let go of what is not serving you. Just let it be. Focus on what is, and in stressful times, use your breath to remind you to be present. Smell the flowers, kiss your babies. Life is tough for busy women, there is no doubt. But regardless of your circumstances, YOU are the most important, Goddess. Whatever you do, don't forget that.

The Power of Gratitude

We Goddesses believe that in our society we really take our food for granted. Taking a moment during a meal to send out a message of gratitude to whomever or whatever you like - The Universe, The Earth, God, the local farmer who grew your veggies, the chef for preparing it- can only help your digestion and enhance your life. When you take a moment to say thank you, you instantly cultivate a moment of peace within, as you slow down and focus on what is really important. Say your thank yous!

Sanctity of Food As Love

Once you have begun to eat in the ways listed above, your view on food will never be the same. Just as it is a miracle that you are alive, so too is it a miracle that there is gorgeous, nourishing food to keep you alive.

Food and traditions around food are a part of every culture, and always have been. Food brings us closer to the ones we love. The food that you eat should, as often as possible, be prepared with reverence and love, and consumed and enjoyed in the same way. Give your home and your family a gift by always setting your table, and as often as you can, sit with your with your family at meal times and talk about the good things in life. While you are there, take a moment every time to appreciate the beauty and the magic of the dinner table, as you watch your family connect with each other and celebrate their bond over a beautiful, simple meal.

Falling Through The Ice

In recovering from my[5] own personal struggle with fatigue, exhaustion and burnout, a beautiful analogy was explained to me by a man with an amazing and innovative view of health care. Dr. Gordon Hasick is a NUCCA chiropractor and one of my greatest teachers. He has generously agreed to share his analogy with you, Goddess, and we are forever grateful for his wisdom.

The Building Foundations of Personal Health
by Dr. Gordon Hasick, DC

When it comes to staying healthy, you would think that it would be easy. It would be natural. We now have advanced healing technologies and health care facilities to help us stay healthier and in some ways, we are.

*Recently, the World Health Organization indicated that a rise of **"chronic"** illnesses is occurring in North America. This offers a significant challenge to our current health care system. The traditional model of health care has worked remarkably well in dealing with acute illness through crisis care, but it does not seem to have the same beneficial effects on chronic, long-standing conditions.*

---

5 Where appropriate, we may refer to ourselves in the singular. This is to show that one of us has had a personal story to share. We do not believe it is necessary to indicate which of us the story is referring to.

With new research constantly emerging and growing consumer demands for alternative answers, wellness or preventative self-care will need to come to the forefront of our health care system. This will likely challenge the old beliefs about health care, as we know it. It seems that now may be the time to respond to the changing health challenges and begin a new approach that will produce more positive long-term healing effects for your well-being.

From a Wellness Conference in Toronto in 1986 the following statement was developed:

"Wellness is more than a concept. It is a way of life, an integrated enjoyable approach to living that emphasizes the importance of achieving "harmony" in all parts of the person; mind, body and spirit. More than an absence of illness, it is a balance among all of the aspects of the person."

With all the newly developed health technology and all this new help, why is there an increase in many chronic long-standing conditions? My clinical experience has revealed the simple common practices, or ***Building Foundations of Personal Health****, are most often overlooked! These are the health creation tools that are simple, cost effective to use and work to support your well-being! These tools are built upon well established principles of basic human physiological needs. They* ***must*** *be met in order to sustain life, let alone good health.*

If we look at the increasing pace of our busy and often stressful lives, our health and well-being could be viewed like ice skating on a deep frozen lake. We need to have ice that is thick enough to carry our weight. In other words, our body needs to be healthy enough to support our activities of daily life "and" the load that we carry day to day needs to be reasonable. As we push our bodies by stressing our systems with such things as poor nutrition, lack of activity, poor air quality and lack of adequate rest, our physiological ice gets thinner and thinner. We then we take on more responsibility, more work, more worry, and stress at a pace of life that is much faster.

The ***"load"*** *that we carry on the* ***thin ice*** *can have some very devastating health consequences. Eventually, if the load is too great and the ice is too thin, we fall through. Our system collapses into disease and often burnout.*

The opposite of stress is not relaxation, but resilience! It is about making sure that the foundation upon which you stand is adaptable and solid!

There are five foundational principles that our health and optimal physiology are built upon. What are needed are tools and practices to enhance your well-being. These principles are the things that build thicker ice and enhance your resilience. In addition to any health care treatment or once you have achieved your desired level of health, these steps help you ***maintain*** *your health. Either way, they must be included in each step along the way.*

We have to earn our health and once we have achieved it, the challenge and responsibility is maintaining it. This is where these principles are foundational. They may seem simplistic and they are. The benefits that are experienced when you attended to them regularly are very significant! The health care choices are endless, but in any situation we need a place to start. Those people that commit to and attend to these foundational principles have consistently enjoyed better health and an improved quality of life.

Why not give them a try?

Air
Water
Rest
Nutrition
Activity

Go Goddess!

One Thing

There is a lot of information in Chapter Two, we know. It was actually hard to choose the best, One Thing for you to try. What we decided on is this: choose one dark green leafy vegetable to buy this week.

Trying something like kale or Swiss Chard accomplishes the essence of this chapter: Taking the time to commit to selecting the most nutrient dense, digestion friendly food you can. Just buy some nice, crispy looking leaves of either kind (organic, if you can find them), hold a leaf in your hand, and strip the stem out of the middle. Then, chop the leafy bits very fine, and just sprinkle them on your salad. Be sure to take the time to chew your salad very well, as the fibre is not digestible. The better you chew it, the more absorbable it will be. These beautiful vegetables give you energy boosting B vitamins for energy and hormone balance, tons of bone building calcium, and good fibre for your colon.

Bonus: One MORE Thing

Ok, if you are ready for more- try this: chew your food to liquid at least once in the day. That's about 30 chews per bite. You need to MAKE the time to do this, but that's the whole point. Respect yourself enough to take the time to SLOWLY eat a meal. Properly chewed food, that can be digested and therefore absorbed more easily will give you energy. Chewing it well first will take the burden off your digestive system, thus conserving your precious energy.

"You are about to embark on a journey down a new path. And here's my advice. Never, ever accept mediocrity posing as convenience. Never, ever accept glitter over substance. Care about what you eat: Absolutely insist that it be delicious and true; and never, ever accept anything less. When you sit down to a real meal, with real food, the body is fed, and having been fed and delighted, the soul is nourished. And only then are you able to become the amazing being you were born to be!"

Jude Blereau, Wholefoods

CHAPTER TWO

Hydrate

I believe that prior to Adam and Eve, water itself held the consciousness of God- that God's intention was put into the medium of water, and that this was used in the creation of Earth and Nature.

-Masaru Emoto

Get Ready...

What are you made of? Yup, just like your mom told you. Water. Not wine, not puppydog tails. You are made of the most vital element on our beautiful planet. Pure water. It's not like this is a shock. It's not like you haven't heard that you need to drink it. So why do you continue to avoid it? Some people won't drink water without some kind of artificial sweetener type drink crystal stirred in. Some people think they get enough if they just eat fruit and vegetables. Some think that the water that comes in their coffee and tea and juice provides enough hydration for their bodies to live on.

Ok, here's the straight goods. You need to drink your water. Stop being babies about it and be Goddesses instead. Yes, you need to drink lots. Most experts recommend drinking at least 2 litres of water a day. We say drink as much as you comfortably can. Your body knows how much is enough if you listen to its cues. No, coffee doesn't count. In fact, coffee is a diuretic, so that means that it pulls water out of your system. For every cup of caffeinated beverage you consume, you must drink an EXTRA glass of water on top of your regular amount.

So let's talk about why.

Get Set...

Well, it's just like anything else we've talked about so far. If you want the absolute best function for your gorgeous Goddess body, then you have to give it what it needs. And it needs water. And not just any kind of water, either. The best water for a human body is pure spring water. Spring water contains essential minerals that help water absorb into your system. Tap water often contains chlorine and fluoride, both of which bind with the iodine that your body needs for your thyroid to function properly, and flushes that iodine out of your system. If your thyroid doesn't get enough iodine, then its function slows, and your metabolism slows too. When your metabolism slows down, you feel sluggish, tired, and it may be hard for you to shed the extra pounds you are carrying.

Water also helps us detoxify pollutants from our system, like flushing your car's lines out when you take it to the mechanic.

There are foods that help hydrate us as well. Cucumber, coconut, celery, grapes and many other fruits contain extra water that will help keep our system humming. Try adding some cucumbers and mint leaves to a tall pitcher of cool spring water on a hot summer day and see how it makes you feel...

So, Goddess, remember: the rule of thumb with water is the same as with your food. Drink only the best within your means. If you can find really good quality spring water, then that is your best bet. The minerals in it will help the water absorb into your cells. At the very least, please try to filter out the chlorine and fluoride and medicinal drugs that circulate through your city's water supply. There are many good resources on the internet that discuss water filtration systems. Remember this, though - distilled water and reverse osmosis water are pure, but they contain no minerals at all to help your water absorb. Adding a small pinch of Celtic Sea Salt or Himalayan Rock Salt to your water bottle will help you balance your minerals if you must consume water that has none.

Buy yourself a funky, stainless steel water bottle and keep it filled. You will be amazed how good you feel when you give your body what it needs.

Oh yah, and don't worry about the peeing thing. Yes, when you increase your good quality water consumption, you may pee more at first. But this is a natural way of your body cleansing toxins out of your system. If your water contains the minerals it needs to help it absorb, instead of it passing right through you, it will absorb into your cells. Be patient with your body. Let it balance. If you give it what it needs, it will balance in time.

Go Goddess!

One Thing

Your One Thing for this chapter is to commit to drinking at least one litre of water a day. As we said, you should ultimately have two. If you are someone that relies on sugary pop or juice, swap at least one glass of the sweet stuff for a glass of clear, beautiful, energy giving water, and then, stop, and really pay attention to how you feel once you have sipped it. A lot of people notice that they have more energy, less odd hunger pains, less pain in joints and muscles, and a clear, sharp brain. A hydrated body is a beautiful body. Add a bit of lemon to it, or cucumber, or even berries- you will be nourishing your body even further. If you close your eyes and sip, it will feel like you are at the spa!!

CHAPTER THREE

Breathe

I took a deep breath and listened to the old bray of my heart. I am. I am. I am.

–Sylvia Plath

Breathe

Get Ready...

Of course we know you know how to breathe...

But do you really? The gift of proper breath is one of the most amazing things you can do for yourself. Believe it or not, there is a right and a wrong way to breathe.

If you watch a baby breathing while they sleep, you will notice that their whole bodies move, as their tummies rise on the inhalation and fall on the exhalation. Breathing this way puts them in a deep state of relaxation and helps them sleep like, well, babies.

So how do we breathe? Well, it seems that as we age, we forget this most important skill. We have adapted our breath to accommodate our high stress lifestyles. When we are in a situation that is stressful, we breathe the opposite to babies - our stomachs suck in on the inhalation and push out on the exhalation. When we breathe this way, we signal to our body, once again, that that tiger is after us. As soon as we rise our shoulders and suck our stomachs in with the breath, adrenaline begins to pump, and fight or flight kicks in.

Get Set...

Ok Goddess, so why should you concentrate on changing how your breath works? Well, first because, just like a baby, when you breathe a belly breath, the same thing that happens to babies, happens to you - a deep state of relaxation begins to set in. Blood pressure drops, and your happy chemicals like serotonin begin to kick in. Basically, when you breathe properly, you signal to your body that all is well. No more adrenaline, no more stress. Will you do this all the time? Of course not. But here's the trick: every time you are stuck in traffic, or late for an interview or frustrated with the kids, try to make it a habit to become aware of if you are holding your breath. You probably are. Or at the very least, your breathing is shallow and rapid, your shoulders possibly moving up and down. As soon as you notice you are doing this, stop and change gears.

Take a moment. Remember, this whole book is about putting yourself first. So breeeeeeeaaaathe. Properly. Even just a couple of times. Put your hands on your belly and do the "One Thing" on the next page.

Go Goddess!

One Thing

- Blow your stressed out air out through your mouth like you are blowing through a straw. Take a minute to just let go of whatever is not serving you in Goddessdom.
- Then place your hands on your belly. Allow your belly to fill up like a balloon, slowly. Breathe this breath through your nose, for about a count of 4.
- If you like, you could hold your breath now for a count of seven.
- Then release, through your mouth again, like blowing through a straw, for a count of eight.
- Do this four times. You can do this as an exercise, twice a day if you like.
- At the very least, do it when you know you need it. Even if you just do a proper breath once, it is enough to break the stress pattern you are in, slow you down a minute, and bring your attention back to where it belongs - the present moment (where all is always well).

Before you go to sleep at night, begin to be aware of the sound of your breath, as it moves in and out through your nose. Focus on the sound as you place your hands on your belly, feeling your stomach rise as you inhale and fall as you exhale. When you feel your mind wandering (to shopping lists, to do lists) just bring your attention back to the sound of your breath. And then take a moment to be grateful for the air you breathe and the miracle that your body gives you this gift of breath every day, without you even having to think about it. So give it a gift back: beautiful, blissful belly breaths!

CHAPTER FOUR

Joyful Movement

There are short-cuts to happiness,
and dancing is one of them.

~Vicki Baum

Joyful Movement

Get Ready...

Moving your body should always be joyful.

This idea that society has that you have to slap your iPod on, stick a tabloid magazine in front of you to relieve the boredom or jump on a stair climber machine is so very joyless. It was, in fact, very hard to find a really beautiful, inspiring quote for the beginning of this chapter. Most quotes on exercise that we found were along this vein: "Exercise is a dirty word. When I say it, I want to wash my mouth out with chocolate." Cartoonist Charles Schulz said that. Funny? Sure. Sad? Absolutely. Our modern society has a particularly warped idea of what movement is supposed to be for humans. Movement, in fact, is the most natural thing that we, as animals, do. The trouble is not with exercise, but with the lack of respect our society gives the human form and the fact that due to that lack of respect, everything we do has been made to be more convenient, and in turn, less dynamic. Sitting still for hours is easy. Riding an escalator is easy. Driving is easy. But walking, dancing, lifting... our society sees these things as archaic, as time consuming and as something that injures the body, causing pain.

When we do jump on a stair climber or treadmill, we do it to get our exercise out of the way, so we can feel justified in sitting for another eight hours in a stuffy building in front of a computer. The motivation to move does not come from a place of joy - just obligation. Goddess, it doesn't have to be this way.

The Universe has created our bodies to be dynamic, sexy, fluid and beautiful. Regardless of our shape and size, if we are relatively able people, we are all capable of moving our bodies in ways that bring us as much joy as those chocolate brownies do. When you respect yourself deeply, you know that moving your body means a strong heart, strong bones and muscles, and the ability to adapt to the changing circumstances life throws our way every day.

We are creatures that were born to move!

Sitting at a computer or in a minivan for eight hours simply does not maximize our potential! Create joy when you move, Goddess. Here's how.

Get Set...

Conscious movement comes from a place of resilience and balance. When we move, even in a dynamic fashion, we need to always remember to maintain an element of fluidity within our body. What that means is, dear Goddess, the most powerful movement, the kind that is beneficial and supportive to your body, is done from a place of peace and joy.

We are conditioned to think of strength as the tensing and flexing of bulky muscle, where in fact, it is that kind of tension and rigidity that causes injury and instability within your frame and your mind.

You have real strength within you right now- if only you would let yourself go enough to find it, and feel it.

We spend so much of our energy and internal strength carrying around stresses and the heavy weight of the problems of others. Why do we think this is our responsibility? What does worrying do? We can never worry our way out of a problem. So why spend our precious energy trying? Instead, why not take a beautiful, inspired, full breath, and slowly, joyfully, begin to mooooooove.....

Steps to Relaxing Movement

You know, many books have been written by seriously wise sages on the amazing benefits of yoga. Just so we're all clear, that's not what this book is. That said, the Goddess needs gentle, relaxing movement to help her refresh her mind, relax her tired muscles, and get her energy flowing, especially after extremely stressful days. We believe that yoga is such a great fit for this. You can always delve deeper into the ancient art of yoga- take a class, read a book, become an instructor even. But for now, Goddess, here are some steps that include simple, lovely movement that has its roots in yoga. Of course, you should always chat with a health care professional before trying any new exercise.

- Find a quiet place where you have enough room to move around freely.
- Turn down the lights, light a candle, put on your favorite music. Sometimes, just a simple drum beat works well- very tribal, very primal.
- Begin in a seated position, and take just a minute, with your hands at your heart, to slow your mind down.
- Begin to focus on the sound of your breath, as it moves easily in and out through your nose.
- When you feel that you have slowed your heart down enough that your mind begins to feel like it has enough space in it to let in gentle, healing energy, come to a standing position.
- Slowly, softly, begin to sway. Use your hips and gently rock, side to side.
- When the swaying begins to feel natural, bend your knees slightly, and get your body rocking a little more.

- Begin to add your arms in, swing them gently, side to side, moving them up high, above your head, down low, side to side - whatever feels comfortable and natural.

- This series of movement should begin to get your heart beating just a little faster. Take a moment and revel in this experience - this freeing, soft, fluid movement. What feelings are you experiencing? Do you want to laugh? Cry? Just be with the feelings and the movement. Then begin to slow it down.

- Once your body has come to a standstill, bring your hands in prayer position to your heart again. Take a moment to get centered, listening to the sound of your breath, feeling your heart.

- When you feel ready, sweep your hands out to either side, making a circle, until they reach straight above your head. Allow your palms to meet. Breathe in.

- In prayer position, draw your hands straight down from above your head, in a straight line, to your heart again. Breathe out as you do this.

- Repeat this simple movement as many times as you like. When you are ready, you will change it up a bit. Instead of drawing your hands down to your heart, take them out from above your head, sweeping them down, as if you were a bird, diving with its wings straight out to the side. Bend forward as you do this, and allow your hands to meet your feet, or knees, or whatever you can reach. Be sure to bend your knees a bit, to protect your back.

- When you are bent right over, place your hands on the floor, and step back, so that you are prone - legs out straight behind you, toes curled under, hands flat on the ground by your face, arms bent and hugged to your side, nose to the ground. Take a moment to breathe.

- Inhale, and as you exhale, push your midsection up, letting your behind point to the sky - hands and feet are on the floor, and your body forms a triangle, with the floor at the bottom. In yoga, this position is called "Downward Facing Dog". Bend your knees slightly, and work at slowly letting your heels drop towards the floor. The balls of your feet stay anchored on the ground. Keep your arms relatively straight, being careful to keep a little bend in your elbows- you want to always be respectful of your joints. Be here, with your back flat, your neck straight with your spine, and breathe for about 5 breaths. To come out, slowly step your feet in, stand up slowly and sweep your arms back to prayer position at your heart.

- Have a seat, Goddess. Feel your beautiful body planted firmly on the earth. Remember at this time that you are so connected to the Earth- born of it, made of it. Bend your knees and stick your feet out to the left. Place your left hand on your right knee, and inhale. Gently twist your spine to the right, exhaling as you do. Be gentle! Only twist as far as you can, and hold as long as is comfortable - a few breaths. Repeat on the other side.

- Come out of the twist, and scoot your bum up against a wall.

- Lying flat on your back, keep your bum touching the wall and slide your legs straight up the wall. Allow your arms to drop to your sides, palms up. Feel free to place a pillow or two under your pelvis if it feels good. Be here, and breathe. This pose should not be done if you are menstruating or have high blood pressure. To come out, slide your legs down, and roll to your side, being careful to slowly rise to a sitting position. Use your top hand to help you up.

- Finally, get comfy. Grab a blanket and lie flat on your back, legs out straight. Go ahead and place a pillow under your knees, should you need it. Allow your hands to fall to your sides, palms up. Allow your legs to relax- your feet will fall out to the sides. Be here and breathe, focussing on the gentle sound of your breath. Your belly will rise as you inhale and fall as you exhale.

Don't worry if this doesn't happen for you right away. Just enjoy the feeling of breathing. With every breath, allow yourself to be in a place of release. Let go of anything that doesn't serve you in the present moment. Be mindful of if you are clenching your jaw, frowning, tightening your tummy unconsciously... just allow everything to let go. When you let go of everything you don't need - jealousy, worry, anger, sadness, judgement - there is only love and healing energy left. When you are really still, really, really quiet, existing only for the present moment, you are at one with the healing energies of the Universe.

Allow this to become your new reality.

Feel yourself fill with love, and rejoice in it.

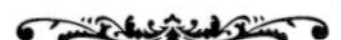

Go Goddess!

One Thing

We realize, Goddess, that all the steps above may seem a little daunting at first. That's ok! To make things less complicated, go ahead and just start by taking a moment to centre yourself, and then, when you are ready, begin to just rock your hips from side to side, swaying to your favorite music. Close your eyes and just let your body go. Even just doing this, for five, ten minutes a day does some amazing things:

- Raises your heart rate, burns calories, strengthens your heart.
- Frees the powerful female energy that is stuck in your pelvic region and allows joy to flow freely.
- Allows you to experience the sensation of freedom - of dancing for no one but yourself.

The more willing you are to surrender to the energy within you, the more power can flow through you.

-Shakti Gawain

CHAPTER FIVE

The Importance of SPA

Tension is who you think you should be. Relaxation is who you are.

~Chinese Proverb

*

There must be quite a few things that a hot bath won't cure, but I don't know many of them.

~Sylvia Plath

SPA

Get Ready…

Ahhhh, SPA. Our favorite three letters in one beautiful little word. For the Goddess, spa has come to mean three things:

S: Self Care

P: Protecting My Reserves

A: Acknowledging my right to deserve to be pampered

It's time to move a little deeper inside and look at how to care for you on a body-mind level.

Respecting the Goddess Within

Many of us have mothers who grew up in an era where the way they defined themselves as women was directly related to how busy they could stay. We have all met these women. In fact, heck, maybe some of us ARE these women. They are constantly moving, being busy doing lots of things at once and sometimes busying themselves with nothing in particular. These are the women who say things like, "I'll sleep when I'm dead" or, when they come to your house for dinner, they are the first to hop up, clear the dishes and begin scrubbing your kitchen while everyone else relaxes with a glass of wine. These are the women who, if they DID in fact stop, would find themselves face to face with their own, very real issues and this scares them. They are also the women whose egos define them by how much they can do for others in the shortest amount of time.

Maybe you are one of these women. Or, you could also be a woman who just hasn't quite realized the vital importance of taking some regenerative time for herself. Either way, this chapter is for you, Goddess, as it will help guide you to a place where you can accept that doing nothing IS doing something. And something very important at that.

Most women in our society think of SPA as an extravagance. Spas themselves are very expensive and, unless you are in a wedding party, cater to the elite. That said though, SPA does not have to mean $200 facials or retreats in the mountains (ooohhh, as lovely as those things are).

SPA can mean for you whatever it takes to achieve body-mind balance. At the very least, it should mean taking even ten minutes every day to turn your mind inwards, slowing down your thoughts and your body and allowing the doors to your cells to open so that restorative energy can flood in.

You are worth it, Dearest Goddess. Self care will make you someone YOU can live with- a better human being, a gentler mother, a more motivated worker, a more understanding and patient partner. When you take time for yourself and take a few minutes to acknowledge and show respect to your inner Goddess, you maintain a connection between your body, your mind and your spirit. This internal, quiet place is your solace. The place you can go to regenerate and renew whenever you are feeling low, feeling alone, feeling exhausted. It is always there for you, you just need to slow down and take the time to find it and spend time there.

Get Set...

In case this is a foreign concept to you, here are some basic "how to spa" suggestions:

- Have a bath. It seems simple, but water is a very powerful tool. In fact, at a recent conference we attended, Dr. Andrew Weil said that a spa just isn't a spa unless there is water involved. Lock your door, put on some gentle, soothing music, light a candle and turn off the lights. Add some epsom salts, which are full of muscle relaxing magnesium, grab a nice big glass of lemon water so you stay hydrated. Drop in some lavender essential oil to your bath water and breathe in the blood-pressure lowering aroma.
- Get your favorite stainless steel travel mug, fill it with nurturing herbal tea like Rooibos or Peppermint and go for a slow walk outside. Take your time, listen to your breath, observe nature. Become quiet. Slow your thoughts- no lists, no self bad mouthing, no conversation at all. Just stillness and being present. Regard Mother Nature as you walk and think to yourself, "I am all of this, it is me". Notice a flower as

it is blooming, a bird lighting on a tree. Be right with nature and right with the present moment. Take in deep, beautiful belly breaths. Smile.

- Gather the Goddess Group- have a spa night with your dearest, closest girls. Invite a professional esthetician to your home and have her do everyone's toes. Have a massage therapist give mini massages. Bring out big bowls and fill them with warm water, flower petals, floating candles and peppermint. Make Goddess crowns out of willow branches and decorate them like you were six years old. Soak feet, paint toes, light candles, laugh, eat, dance, indulge. Honor your friends with simple, loving gestures and allow them to do the same for you. Celebrate the awesome power of women all together.

- Invite ritual into your life. Plan a bed time routine that allows you to pamper yourself and remind you of your power as Goddess. Light your candle, set it in the west, and surround it with whatever is important to you, kind of like an alter for your spirit- pictures, crystals, books, whatever is sacred just to you. Get your best, most soul enriching book ready, have your bath, do ten minutes of Goddess Movement, read, then breathe. Put on your most luxurious night wear, and slip into clean sheets. Do your belly breaths and drift off to sleep.......

Go Goddess!

One Thing

To properly SPA, one must remember the three things we said the letters mean at the start of this chapter. So, your one thing today is to do the "A"- acknowledge your right to deserve to be pampered. When we spa, there is no guilt, no thinking about your pile of paper at work, what your children are doing or how your partner's day was more stressful than yours. Spa comes from a place of joy, always. So to complete your One Thing, do the following:

- turn off your cell phone
- take 10 minutes or more when you know you will not be interrupted
- choose to do whatever feels restorative, restful, and a little indulgent for those ten minutes- a walk, a bath, a massage...
- Think of nothing else while you are SPA-ing. Just be in the moment and breathe. If you find that your mind is wandering to a place of guilt, say the following mantra:

"I acknowledge my right to deserve to be pampered. By taking time to rest and restore my body and mind, I am protecting my energy reserves, and giving myself the gift of self care and self love. I am whole."

Part Two:

Care of the Goddess Spirit

CHAPTER SIX

Inspiration

Without inspiration the best powers of the mind remain dormant, they are a fuel in us which needs to be ignited with sparks.

- Johann Gottfried Von Herder

Inspiration

Get Ready...

Don't skip over this part, Goddess!

It may seem fluffy, but this is important stuff. So hang in there, and indulge us....

There are days when all of us feel completely uninspired.... there are days where the hours seem to just melt into each other.... when our drive and motivation are in the toilet. We have all felt this way. Feeling utterly UNinspired is utterly depressing. Sometimes, when we are emotionally exhausted, the last thing we could ever imagine feeling is inspired. Or even wanting to feel inspired. Why is inspiration important? Because it is the spark plug that ignites joy.

We can experience inspiration on many levels. On the grandest, when we are inspired, we are completely in the present moment and fully connected to the universal power. This power has helped many great people do amazing things for humanity- Picasso, Austen, Mozart, Einstein, Angelou, Coltraine, Ghandi- all did what they did for our world because of inspiration.

Our world would be a very different place without these people and the inspiration that drove them to complete their life's work. And fair enough. For a mom of four kids, however, who works a full time job, cleans a house and volunteers at her children's school in her spare time, inspiration can have another function entirely. And we are not saying here, that if you **are** this mom, you won't go on to create a masterpiece that changes the face of history as we know it- of course you can, and many others have- but from a practical standpoint, let us introduce you to another way to use inspiration.

In this crazy, busy world, we all use tools to help us cope with the stresses of life. Some of us use things like yoga and deep breathing and that's good, and some of us use wine and antidepressants. Sometimes the latter is a tool that your doctor feels is medically necessary. And that's ok. But antidepressants, wine or yoga or not, what is missing when we are feeling over our heads, drowning in exhaustion and misery for our present circumstances, is a sense of joy- of utter freedom, happiness and contentment for where we are right at that moment. But joy won't just happen if there isn't space for it to grow.

Inspiration allows us to create a space in our world where we can put a bucket of joy and let it simmer, even if we are not ready to use it. What inspires you literally gets you from moment to moment in your day. If your day consists of being a taxi for your children, or commuting to work for hours on a stinky, crowded bus, then what inspires you can make the drearier parts of your day more manageable. Kinda like wine, but without the hangover. The little things that bring you inspiration to get from one moment to the next are also the things that remind you who YOU are as a woman.

Get Set...

Here's an example. I spend a lot of time sitting in vehicles, dropping children off at various engagements. There is a certain group of songs on my iPod that, when played, transport me a little bit away from where I currently exist. Is this escapism? Maybe. But it is also a way for me to remember my own feelings. Every time one of my favorite songs is played, I am filled with emotions that belong, uniquely, to me. When I am feeling the overwhelming sensation that I am Mom, and Mom alone, I put on those tunes and sing at the top of my lungs. I experience the feelings and sensations the songs evoke in me as they arrive and I am faithfully reminded that I- me, the woman inside the mom- am still here, feeling these feelings, experiencing this music that I love so much and being in the moment as the music is played. When the songs are over, I feel refreshed, and back on centre. If I don't, I play the songs again.

Many things do this for us- remind us of our loves, our passions, our raisons d'être. When we continually remind ourselves of these things, the little space inside, where the bucket of joy is sitting, waiting, begins to grow. As we continue to experience this kind of inspiration - first using it as a coping tool, and later as our way of finding our centre - the joy grows, and eventually, it becomes free flowing.

The trick here, when you are feeling utterly slovenly and down in the dumps, is to make the conscious, respectful choice for your spirit to use inspiration to get you through your day, instead of making a choice that feeds only your ego - like a bag of licorice with a heavy dose of guilt on top. Choosing inspiration puts positive energy in your joy bucket. The guilt sucks your energy away.

As our respect for who we are as women is fostered and nurtured, so too is joy. When we begin to experience joy regularly, a powerful circle is created. Unbridled joy paves the way, then, for inspiration in the larger sense of the word.

And THAT is when we are able to create true change. First in ourselves, and over time, in the rest of the world.

Go Goddess!

One Thing

So you can really get the gist of this part of the book, we have offered up for you OUR list of things that inspire us in different ways- the things that move us to create and the things that bring us back to centre. Once you have read through ours, give yourself a Goddess Gift and take the time to do the same thing for you in the blank chart we have provided.

Inspires me to do great things	Inspires me to get through my day
My family, and the legacy I can leave for my kids.	When my daughters bring me a work of art that is made for me.
Women- watching your fierce determination, struggles, peacefulness, and unconditional love.	Looking forward to a girls night in... paint toes, drink a great glass of wine, laugh together.

Inspires me to do great things	**Inspires me to get through my day**
Mother Nature- the Rocky Mountains, the Pacific Ocean, the trees, the animals- everything.	Fresh flowers on my kitchen table.
Authors who are mothers-busy, but fearless enough, and centred enough, to write books that entertain millions.	Reading a great book in a hot bath.
My best girls. They never laugh at my ideas, remind me that I can do anything.	A good phone chat with a girlfriend.
Food. Growing it, working with it, tasting it, teaching about it, loving it.	Throwing a dinner party, cooking for and serving my friends. A really lovely cup of tea.
The process of writing.	The smell of books and coffee at my favorite book store.
The way someone looks when something we have taught them starts to make sense-the light goes on!	Listening to my favorite tunes.

Your Own Inspiration Chart

What Inspires You?

To get through your day	To do great things

CHAPTER SEVEN

Spirit

It isn't until you come to a spiritual understanding of who you are - not necessarily a religious feeling, but deep down, the spirit within - that you can begin to take control.

- Oprah Winfrey

Spririt

Get Ready...

Having fun so far, Goddess? We are!

In the previous chapters, we provided you with the tools to be able to nourish and strengthen your body. Now that you have the hang of that, Goddess, we know you are ready for the really exciting stuff. Now it is time to use what you have learned about yourself and dive a little deeper into the Goddess Potential! Think of this chapter and the ones that follow, as a promise to yourself. Take our information within and then begin to commit to arriving at a place where you understand your own worth, where you embrace the Divine Feminine and can wield that power of self love to heal the world.

A word of caution: only begin this next step if you are sure you are fortified enough to be able to begin to give to others, without sacrificing your own well being.

Strength of spirit takes courage, and courage takes energy. So, be honest with yourself. If you are not feeling yet like you are ready for these next steps, go back in the book and work on whatever area you feel needs attention. You will know when you are ready.

The Divine Feminine

We are certain this term has many meanings but we would like to redefine it as it pertains to the Goddess Lifestyle. To use the term "Divine Feminine" means an acceptance that there is as much divinity in being female and all that is particular to being female, as there is in being male.

There is an unspoken feeling out there that there is somehow something inherently inadequate about being female. Like the wires weren't hooked up properly and only half the lights are blinking. That there is something faulty with the more typical attributes of being feminine, like being emotional, sensitive, protective, curvy, soft.

The Goddess knows that it is time we acknowledged the fact that we are not a mistake. All that is uniquely feminine is Divinely inspired by the Universe (and therefore vital to all life) just as water and air are. Just as our magnificent male counterparts, we too are God's gifts to the Universe. And it's about time we acted like it!

Get Set...

There are three important stops on this journey:

1) Embrace the Goddess Temple and Spirit.

2) Honour yourself by always asking the "Divine Question".

3) Seek the Joy.

Embrace

So here's a thought, fellow Goddesses. If we as women did not spend our time thinking about our weight, the cheesecake we had at lunch, the size of our thighs, or how overly sensitive we were with our spouse, what could we accomplish with all that spare time and brain power? You may think that you don't spend a lot of time on these trivial negative thoughts, but if you really think about it, you will see what time thieves thoughts like these really are.

In the morning when you get dressed, we bet you say at least one wayward remark to yourself about your belly, your butt or the flesh on your arms. How about when you do your makeup? A zit, a wrinkle, a too big nose. Now, there's the hair of course- too thin, too thick, too curly, too straight.

Then we have to tackle breakfast! You'd love that sweet danish but you're supposed to have the two boring poached eggs, so you wrestle with yourself until you walk out of the house on nothing but coffee or the other extreme- TWO danishes, instead. Then you arrive at work and your boss sent you such a scathing email that you burst into tears. Embarrassed by your emotions, you chastise yourself for not having better self control.

Yah...so maybe you spend a little more time on the subject than you thought! And it's only 9 a.m.! So what does this have to do with the daunting topic of Spirituality? Well, the brand of spiritual connectedness we are talking about in this book has nothing to do with an organized religion or a belief in a particular deity. This is literally about your "spirit" as a female entity. No religion or spiritual belief system can ever penetrate your soul if you don't connect **to** your soul, your *self.* So that is what we are talking about. Understanding your own worth and beauty and therefore falling madly in love with yourself, body and soul.

So how do you arrive at this place where you can embrace all that is beautifully and perfectly yours? The journey begins with one key understanding and here it is. Are you ready for it?

You didn't make yourself.

You are a magnificent creature capable of many amazing feats, but the one thing you didn't do was create yourself. It's all well and fine to be humble or self deprecating out of politeness when you are fussing over something that you made, but **you** didn't make **you**.

Look, whether you are a science nut or into the more esoteric, either an all powerful being or an all powerful natural force fought the odds and created you. Anyone who has had trouble conceiving a child knows what a miracle it is that humans even exist. When you know the science of reproduction and you understand that the odds were stacked against you even coming into the world in the first place, it makes it pretty hard to sit there and complain. A Goddess knows that her existence is a gift, both to her soul and to the world. She had nothing to do with the creating of her life, and therefore self depreciation is an inappropriate emotion. Thankfulness and awe for the artist's ability would be more in tune.

What if you don't really care for the handiwork? Well, especially if you do believe in a higher power, why do we always think that that power was successful in every way except our female body or our feminine psyche? Why do we not include them in our cache of personal gifts like our beautiful singing voice and our patience? Why do we say " Thank you God for the flowers and the trees and the butterflies...too bad you went wrong with my thighs!?". No... there is purpose in our feminine traits and our very particular female bodies.

Let's look at the issue of our bodies for a moment, as it seems to be the bitter plague of the female existence. We spend so much time at war with this apparatus that has been specifically created for our experience here.

Your body has a wisdom of its own you know, Goddess. It's not simply a "soul suit" or a random arrangement of genes. It expands and contracts, grows strong and grows weary and sometimes, if we really won't listen to its subtler warnings, it becomes ill.

Why is stress becoming the number one killer in North America? Because our bodies RESPOND to emotion, to our soul.

Often, when we are stressed, our body puts on weight, both through increasing our need for eating and also through slowing of the metabolism through the thyroid. The brilliant wisdom of our innate intelligence understands that high amounts of stress require added fat to protect organs that might otherwise become damaged by a good rip in the gut from a saber tooth tiger. Huh, you say? Well, when we are stressed, our body is programmed with ancient wisdom that tells it that stress equals becoming someone's dinner, not that stress equals your kid spilled his sippy cup contents on your Blackberry, or that the high demands of your successful business are stressing you out. Still confused? Our point is, like we mentioned in the "Nourish" Chapter, your body is like that faithful dog protecting us from harm and loving us even when we ignore it, chastise it or are disappointed in it.

Could it be possible that, with extra weight, the body is trying to protect the soul from the harm of the stresses that we choose to make inherent to our lives?

Could your beautiful body be trying to make itself larger, to be stronger, or to create a barrier (fat) between our very soul and our environment?

Could fat be more than just a physiological let-down? Could our bodies be that wise?

If so, what would happen if we **blessed** our body for its wonderful wisdom and for its inherent knowing that we are perhaps not choosing any other methods of protecting our well being. Even if we still take it for granted, our body, like that ever faithful dog, takes on the occupation of survival for no other thanks than our resentment and desire to change it.

So what if we resigned, or committed ourselves to not focussing obsessively on changing it? In this society, we have this fear that if we accept ourselves as we are and we somehow find happiness, we will become slovenly creatures that never strive for anything greater and we will lay on the couch for the rest of our lives and die of obesity. Well, we have news for you, Goddess. Many women are joylessly resenting themselves and are STILL lying on the couch and dying of obesity anyway!!

Then there is the other extreme, where we deny ourselves our pleasures and put our bodies though punishing, joyless exercise regimes that may bring svelte waistlines but no joy – or only brings the kind of joy that would disappear if we missed a few workouts and gained a few pounds back. No joy at all, really.

How do we behave towards people and things that we love and adore, say a child or a pet? Typically, we shower that child or pet with love and attention, we see to their needs to the best of our abilities, we make tough choices on their behalf to keep them safe and we constantly strive to make them feel precious and loved no matter how many mistakes we may make with them. Generally, barring any major emotional dysfunction, we don't try to kill them with Twinkies. And typically, we don't say things like, "Ok son, when you lose another 25 pounds, I will love you. Until then, you're on your own. Here's a Mr. Big."

So our theory is that if we could reach a place of tender love for ourselves NOW, we may actually make more loving choices for ourselves, like we would for that child or that dog. Perhaps becoming thinner is part of that love, perhaps it's not. But being healthier certainly is. And being loving, gentle, forgiving, kind and GRATEFUL to and for ourselves most definitely should be. Isn't that what we strive for in our other personal relationships? Why? Why do we strive to be more loving, gentle, forgiving and kind to our children, our spouses, our mothers and our best friends? Because it makes life more enJOYable of course...hmmm...there's that little word again...JOY! So wouldn't it be more enjoyable to treat yourself the same way?

Here is a mantra for you to say to yourself when you need some reminding about the awesomeness of your physical form.

My body is a perfect instrument, calibrated perfectly at all times, unfailingly communicating truth to me every minute of the day, and when I choose to listen to it, I will not only achieve physical balance but I will reach true enlightenment with greater ease.

And what of our female emotions? You know what we mean Goddess – in comparison to men we seem so much more complicated, our decisions and courses of action so wrapped up in our emotions and our feelings.

It is easy in this world to feel that these traits are a failing of some kind, but truly embracing yourself as a Goddess means accepting that, like our curvy bodies, our emotions are divinely inspired.

WE WERE MADE THIS WAY AND WE HAVE PURPOSE!

Our emotional souls are nothing less than our God given Source of Power. Our job here is to pay attention to our vast pool of emotions and then draw healing waters from them, all the while being ever vigilant that we are not drowned by them.

As was told to Spiderman (so says my wise, 11 year old son), with great power comes great responsibility. The sheer depth and breadth of our emotional arsenal is a gift to this universe and it is time to respect the gift. It is time to learn to understand the gift and how to honour it.

Honour

Now that you understand your own divinity – your own **worth** both physically and emotionally, how do you celebrate it? How do you keep this knowledge at the center of your daily life so that you become a powerful force? Well Goddess, the answer is that you commit to being honourable to your Self. And you honour your Self with Joy. The most important skill to be learned is how to constantly assess if what you are doing, feeling, eating, breathing is *honourable* to your divine origin.

There is a simple question that you must ask yourself at all times and if the answer to this question is not " it brings me joy" then you need to re-calibrate.

The Divine Question is: " How does this serve me?"

It sounds so Goddessy doesn't it? It's a delicious question and it makes you feel slightly princessy. But make no mistake, this is not a frivolous, indulgent question! All that you choose to spend your precious reserves on must answer this question in a satisfying way or you are wasting your time. Let's put it into practice:

Get Set...

The Divine Question

Here are a few examples of situations where you would apply the Divine Question in order to remind your Self of how to honour your beautiful, Goddessy nature.

Situation: I am doing my hair and it won't lay flat and I start to berate myself because I don't look like the girl on the cover of Cosmo.

Divine Question: How does this serve me?

Divine Answer: It doesn't. It brings me pain, pain of not being "perfect", it brings me frustration with what I have naturally been given and it make me feel ungrateful and dissatisfied. So now that I know that the comment is not bringing me joy, I can choose again. I find a comment that will serve me with JOY instead of pain, frustration, ungrateful and dissatisfied. I choose to say, "I am a Goddess – I don't need my bangs to lay flat to be a Goddess", and then I blow myself a kiss in the mirror.

Situation: My husband is making me so angry and and I just want to scream at him for 7 hours straight!

Divine Question: How does this serve me?

Divine Answer: Well, the anger is serving me by signaling to me that I am not joyous about something - this is important - but holding on to that anger is doing nothing for me. It's a huge weight on my shoulders to carry such an emotion around with me. I am a Goddess and I have no time for that. I need to choose again. I will choose to tell him what I need him to know and nothing else, no name calling, no past-reminding and no apologizing for how I feel. I will listen to his response and then I'll get on with my life, regardless of his answer. Life is too short to be angry for too long!

Situation: I am upset because I was given terrible service by that waitress!!

Divine Question: How does this serve me?

Divine Answer: I could hold on to this frustration all day long and let it carry into my other activities, but I am a Goddess and that just wouldn't do. I must seek the joy – I think I will decide that it's really not worth my precious time to be mad for long – maybe she had a bad day and I will forgive her. Then I can take it off my plate – so to speak! That serves me best this time.

Situation: My friend has betrayed my trust and I am devastated and I want to cry all day.

Divine Question: How does this serve me?

Divine Answer: I honor my sadness – it serves me well to cry and be cathartic with this emotion. I will allow myself to feel its intensity and grieve. But then I will let it go because it does not serve me to feel this way for long – only long enough to process the emotion. It serves me to forgive her and myself and then seek the light in the situation. The light is where the purpose of this lesson lies and it is where I will find the joy again.

Situation: I want that gorgeous fabulous piece of cake in the bakery window – the one with the buttercream icing and the strawberries!!!

Divine Question: How does this serve me?

Divine Answer: It may serve me quite a few calories, but it's too luscious an experience to pass on! I will order myself a piece. I will sit in meditation as I eat it and I will enjoy every bite with no guilt or remorse. I will pay attention to when I have had enough because it would be a shame to let something so delicious make me feel ill. I will stop eating when I am full and save it for another time or leave it on the plate. I will then choose a beautiful salad and high fibre meal for dinner that will help my body temple process the dessert in the best way for my body. I will have my cake and enjoy it, too! Divine!

Get the idea? You will probably have to put this on pink sticky notes all around your home or have it inscribed on the inside of your contact lenses because it will be hard to remember to check in with yourself at first. We are not primed to do this as women. But commit to practicing it and your life will change in the most dramatic and magical ways. You will begin to discern what feels good to you, what feels like a burden, what is important, and what is not. You will begin to lose that numbness of not knowing or valuing yourself and most of all, you will begin to define what it means to feel joyous!

Of course, sometimes life presents us with even greater challenges such as a terminal illness or death of a loved one. As your Goddess Guides, our greatest challenge in developing this lifestyle was making sure that it stood up to ALL of the experiences that we may encounter in this journey, that it didn't insult those experiences that are more than day to day tribulations, and that it actually offered solace and healing. While we don't want to make light of these kind of situations, we do want to INFUSE them with light, meaning there is ALWAYS room for grace. It is in these times, more than any other, that we must be diligent in asking "How does this serve me?" because therein lies the key to not only surviving tragedy but also giving worth to it.

Asking the Divine Question ensures that the lessons that darkness brings lead you back to the light and, of course, the joy.

Seek the Joy (and find the Mission!)

By "seek the joy" we mean that after you ask yourself the Divine Question, your next commitment must be to find the quickest and fastest route to out-and-out joy. This is vital.

It made you flinch a little to read that didn't it?

A lot of us are taught that life must be difficult for it to be worthwhile, that we must learn to struggle and fight for what we want. Well, if that is comforting to you then believe us, seeking joy will be difficult at first!

The world won't support you to begin with. You must constantly remind yourself, daily, hourly, how amazing you are, because you will be shocked at how easily it will fall out of your head. But mark our words, your thoughts become your reality and after an initial uphill battle, you will suddenly find yourself surrounded with like minded people and supportive situations. The path will begin to rise up to meet you. You will start to see how magical the world really is because you will have left the mire of self loathing behind and chosen a path filled with light and love for the gorgeous, sacred, feminine creature that you are!

And why must you run as fast as you can towards joy? Well firstly, WHY NOT! But secondly, you have to hurdle yourself in that direction because that is your mission. Yes, Goddess, you have a sacred mission here – we all do.

So what is your mission? Well, it could be that you will rule the Northern Hemisphere or that you will raise a child who saves a guy from being hit by a bus or maybe you feel so good about yourself one day that you "smile at the cashier at the grocery store and no one else has that day and she was going to go home and cry herself to sleep but now she's not going to and you single handedly saved another soul from a painful night." All because you have expandable thighs, and you decided they were beautiful instead of hideous and that made you joyful and you paid that forward.

You don't have to go on a humanitarian mission to a war torn country to have a purpose in this life (although we would never discourage this kind of ambition!). You merely have to see that nothing even remotely like this brand of joy can come from a place of loathing.

Only when you find joy can you give it away, and that is all you have to do here.

Your sacred mission is to live in a state of joyousness. That is where your mission begins and God only knows where it will take you!

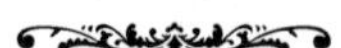

Go Goddess!

One Thing

Here is your "One Thing" to try as you go through the steps to committing to Spiritual Wholeness.

Embrace

Bless your body every day for its obvious and untold wisdom...bless the extra weight, bless the "illness", bless those things that you feel are a burden. They all have a reason, and they all serve to remind you to be good to yourself, and live in joy.

Honour

Do we even have to say it?!

Ask the Divine Question as many times as you can remember to!

Seek The Joy

Choose a joyous option at least once a day, everyday. And then live joyously with your choice.

CHAPTER EIGHT

Get Real, Goddess

I could not, at any age, be content to take my place by the fireside and simply look on. Life was meant to be lived. Curiosity must be kept alive. One must never, for whatever reason, turn (her) back on life.

Eleanor Roosevelt

Get Real, Goddess!

Ok. Admittedly, we have given you a lot to think about.

And the fact of the matter is, we know that even though you now know all this great stuff about how to put yourself first, how to respect your body, how powerful and amazing you truly are, you also still have a mountain of laundry, bills to pay and dishes to wash. We know that life is busy and life can seem fast and, frankly, kind of joyless. We get this, because, as we sit here writing this, our laundry is sitting, neatly folded on the coffee table in the family room, on top of the unpaid bills.

See, Goddess, we are all in this together. That is what is so amazing about this whole process. While you begin to change, and talk to your girlfriends about how you are feeling, they will begin to change too. So sure, the supper dishes are still in the sink, but know this: the point here is not for you to feel more stressed out with the information we have given you, but that, in times of busyness, when life feels overwhelming, you know now to rally the troops and if you need to talk to someone about how life is getting you down, you have great girlfriends who know just what you are going through. And if you don't have any, this is the information age, sister. Hop on the internet and start to chat or blog. There is a world of women out there waiting to talk about how they feel about life. As Ghandi says, "Be the change you wish to see in the world." Start with one thing in this book, and do it tonight. And then tell a girlfriend about it. And then do one more thing tomorrow, and tell your friend about that, too. The laundry will still be there, but you know what? It will get done eventually. Hopefully before your next spa party, or no one will have anywhere to put their champagne cocktails.

Anyway, our point is this. Truly living in a place of joy could happen immediately, if you let it. But our society is not always set up that way and therefore, you need practice. Taking things step by step is the best way to do that. So this week, buy a dark green leafy vegetable you have never used, change over a chemical household cleaning product to something more natural, and choose one day this week where you will have a bath, do a few breaths and get to bed before 10:30. And if that all seems too much, then choose just one of those things to do. The point is that you do them. Start small if you must, and build. Eventually, putting yourself first will become old hat. It will never be a matter of "the laundry or a cup of tea with your feet up". You will instinctively know which one to do first. When you are restored and happy, the laundry will seem so much easier. So much, in fact, that you will choose to do it, and your other mundane tasks from guess where?

A place of joy.

When you are able to feel empowered in your choices, joyfulness naturally follows.

So, no unrealistic expectations here. Just simplicity and love. Make your choices this way, at your own pace, in your own time, joyfully. THAT is what being a Goddess is all about. You first. You heal. And when you heal, the Earth heals. And nothing is more joyful than that.

Part Three:
The Revolution

CHAPTER NINE

The Goddess Revolution

A great revolution in just one single individual will help achieve a change in the destiny of society and, further, will enable a change in the destiny of humankind

–Daisaku Ikeda

The Goddess Revolution

Get Ready...

It's time for a revolution, Goddess.

Some revolutions are big and some are small. Some change one life and some dramatically transform perception and life as we know it. The *Goddess Revolution* intends to do it all – we are aiming for big changes for women and our planet brought about by small changes *you* can make today.

Why a Goddess Revolution and why now? The global imbalances that Mother Earth survives every day, from motherless children in Africa to Western children who go hungry in school lunchrooms, from holes in Mother Nature's magnificent tapestry to losing our connection to the food we serve our families- all of these issues and plenty more are waiting for care and concern, for the restoration in balance through love and nurturing that only a woman is able to foster. This is not a feminist rant. Men have wonderful strengths of their own to contribute. But to this point, they have not been properly balanced with the equal influence of their female counterparts. We are not better than men, we are not even just simply equal to them. We are completely different. Our intuition, our emotions, our inner strength, our sensitivity and our compassion are what allow us to create lasting change in this world.

A woman's truest purpose is to restore balance to the planet through gentle nurturing and fierce love, just as a mother loves her child. But our greatest obstacles are things like ill health, the exhaustion of modern living, our relationships and worries about our appearance and our body. We are worn out and most of us don't have the energy, let alone the time, to fight for the growth of our society or the survival of our planet. Some days we don't even feel like we've given enough quality time to our kids.

Here's the thing. We have been so busy trying to survive our own lives by employing common masculine traits like not crying, not resting, suppressing emotion and burning the candle at both ends. We have never allowed ourselves to surrender to our feminine design. "Surrendering", by the way, does not mean that we need to give anything up or step back in time and undo the progressive work the feminists did. Quite the contrary. By surrendering ourselves to the experience of being a Goddess we simply embrace who we are as a species and just exalt in being women. Goddesses who change our minds, who eat, rest, make love, nurture others with passion and who sometimes cry at silly movies. Women. Still strong, but unapologetic for who we are.

The first purpose of this book is to guide you out of the fog. To help you see that your own health is as important as everybody else's and that the energy you have spent worrying about the shape of your body can be better used cultivating an appreciation for your uniqueness.

So first: take care of yourself. Work with your pain, your exhaustion, your stress. Heal. Recognize that this in and of itself is a process and a journey that begins with love and acceptance of who you are right now. Beginning to even forgive yourself will take some time. But, eventually, and with dedication, you will begin to make small steps towards change.

Then, surrounded in light, go out and be inspired and LIVE. Live joyously. Live full out. Live your one life that you have been given in ways that you never thought possible. Up until now, you've just been too darn tired. And we told you, we get that. But you get it now, too, don't you Goddess? You have the information, so get started. Stop telling yourself that your life is unremarkable. Your life, just as it is right now, is miraculously remarkable. Every one of us has something we can teach, something we can be proud of, and something we can grow from.

Here's a small story. One time, when I was standing in line at Harpo Studios, waiting to see the Oprah Show, I turned to the lady next to me to pass the time. She asked me if this was my first time at the show, and I said "Yes, but it won't be my last- one day I will be a guest". She rolled her eyes and told me she couldn't imagine being a guest on the show. I asked her why and her answer was "I just do not have a remarkable life. There is nothing Oprah would want to talk to me about, and nothing I have to say." I tried to tell her that she was, of course, remarkable, and that she probably had a lot to say, but she just shook her head, and turned away, abruptly ending the conversation. How sad, I thought, that she could live her life, thinking that she had nothing to offer. So afraid of her own power that she would berate herself to a complete stranger.

Let go of the fear.

You can still be a soccer mom, a best friend, a great wife, take care of your house and do things for others every day. You don't need to burn your bra and go all pagan. You can if you like, but mostly, you just need to switch on, wake up, and inhale the joy of life!

In the twentieth century, the call to change for women that came from those great and powerful Goddesses of the Women's Movement fell on a lot of deaf ears. Back then, our society was focussed on things that were based in ego. More money, social status, a better body, a bigger house. Many women in the last century were too busy trying to find their place along side men to give much energy to global causes. We were taught to be tough, to either stay quiet and raise our children or take up arms against our oppressors. Masculine traits like cynicism, bitterness and competitiveness were survival tools that helped up cope, but they got us nowhere.

Now, though, more people, women and men alike, are looking for answers within themselves. They are taking classes and reading better books and being present and taking better care of their children. They are working in earnest to see improvement in their consciousness.

The whole vibration of the Earth, the very consciousness of the planet, is raising. People in general are kinder in this, the twenty first century. We are recycling, we are more spiritual, we are gentler to animals, we are nicer to each other. There is still conflict and darkness out there, but there is also an undercurrent of change right now. A wave of hope that is spreading.

The second purpose of this book is to start a Revolution that will unite women. When we begin to change the way we look at ourselves, the way the world perceives us and the kind of voice we have within it, when we take better care of ourselves and grow in appreciation of our own gifts, we truly step into Goddessness. The Revolution is sparked when we pass this vital information on to another women who needs it, and join together to support and lift each other up.

Get Set

The greatest gift that we as women have is our interconnectedness as "sisters". We naturally lean on one another to get through the difficult times in our lives and we rejoice with each other when life is good. Prior to picking up this book, perhaps your nurturing and giving nature was like an anvil pulling you under that icy water as you tried to give everything to everybody else. Now that you understand about going Goddess, about finding the delicate balance between caring for yourself and caring for others, this inherent womanly gift of giving and nurturing will be resurrected as a source of power that will bring about a better life for you, your sisters, your mothers and your daughters.

When this book was originally published, 111 copies were printed and half were given as gifts to family, friends and clients that we thought could use the information to improve the quality of their lives. The other half of the copies were given to random women, around the world, hoping that the books would find their way to women that needed them.

We want the spirit of this original distribution of *Go Goddess* to stay intact so that every women is gifted this book by another women who cares about her personally or simply as a "sister" Goddess. The transformative power of showing another woman that you care about her and support her is immense, both for the giver and the receiver.

In addition, as one Goddess passes this life preserver to another, more and more women will learn to heal, grow and be filled with joy. It is impossible for the Earth herself not to heal when her human counterparts are freed from the weight they carry. With the skills that stepping into Goddessness teaches us, more and more women will have the energy and the will to do more than merely survive, they will do no less than save the world. It will all start with a simple expression of love from one woman to another.

Go Goddess!

Here is your mission, Goddess. It's not hard but it will change one life at a time on so many levels and it will create a ripple effect that will start with you and perhaps touch another woman, half a world away from you.

Read this book, follow the advice and feel better – begin the healing process for yourself first!

When you are starting to feel better, less stressed and more joyful, take a quite moment to think of a woman that may benefit from Going Goddess. If you can't think of someone, think of a place where women may gather. Consider if it would be possible to simply hand the book to a woman there or if there is a place where you can leave it safely so it can be picked up by someone in need. Perhaps someone at the local YWCA, the park or your workplace could use the support.

It's time now to pass on the wisdom. Remember to keep a copy of *Go Goddess* for yourself to use as a reference and to remind yourself about caring for YOU first, but gift a copy to the woman in your life who needs it. Better yet, as you give it to her, tell her YOUR story – we always fear that we are the only ones experiencing difficulty. When you share your personal journey it empowers both of you, as you lift each other up towards greater change. You will start your very own chain of healing and light and your impact on the world you live in will be extraordinary.

When you have fulfilled you mission of sharing this book and your own amazing story, you will have fully stepped into your own light and power as a Goddess! Little by little, the world will begin to shift and heal and grow and more changes, more opportunities for joyous, empowered living will avail themselves to you and women everywhere.

Start standing where you need to be, Goddess. Take your place in the centre of the Universe, in your power, surrounded by light, love and healing. And then, take a deep breath... and let the joy spread. THIS is the revolution we need. It doesn't come from opposition or anger. It comes from love. From a place of complete acceptance for yourself, for compassion and love for your daughters and sons, for the creatures of the earth, for Mother Earth.

Revolutionize the world with joy, Goddess.

It is your turn!

What are you waiting for?

When a woman has owned her passionate nature, allowing love to flood her heart, her thoughts grow wild and fierce and beautiful. Her juices flow. Her heart expands. She has thrown off crutch and compromise. She has glimpsed the enchanted kingdom, the vast and magical realms of the Goddess within her. Here, all things are transformed. And there is a purpose to this: that the world might be mothered back to a great and glorious state. When a woman conceives her true self, a miracle occurs, and life around her begins again.

Marianne Williamson- A Woman's Worth

CHAPTER TEN

The Recipes

Some people like to paint pictures, or do gardening, or build a boat in the basement. Other people get a tremendous pleasure out of the kitchen, because cooking is just as creative and imaginative an activity as drawing, or wood carving, or music.

– Julia Child

Good Goddess Fare: Joyful Recipes for the Enlightened Woman

Cooking isn't just about putting ingredients together.

And it's not just about finding the best ingredients possible, either. The Goddess knows that cooking is joyful. Julia Child had it right all along.

Here are some recipes that are simple and really nutrient dense. Packed with nutrients, these recipes are supportive to your hormones, boosting to your immunity, balancing to your body and sumptuous to your senses.

With humble gratitude, we share these with you. Know that when we sit down at our dinner tables, you, Goddess, are always in our hearts.

Bon Appetit!

Sumptuous Smoothie

A great way to start your day is with something packed with nutrients, and something that will keep your blood sugar steady for a least a couple of hours. A smoothie is perfect for this.

Ingredients:

2 scoops protein powder or hemp seeds (Protein powder: whey or a veg alternative like *Smoothie Infusion by Vega)*

1 cup frozen berries of your choice

1 handful spinach (you can't even taste it, and it pumps up your nutrient intake significantly)

½ cup almond milk, water or unfiltered apple juice

1 banana (optional)

Water to desired consistency

Method:

Blend in blender til smooth. Feel free to add in the following:

- 1 tbsp flax meal, hemp oil or coconut oil (for good fats for brain function, reducing inflammation and boosting immunity)
- 1 tbsp lecithin (will help you digest fats)

- 1 tbsp wheat germ (very high in the antioxidant Vitamin E, for immunity)
- 1 tbsp oat bran (for soluble fibre which is cholesterol reducing, rids the body of excess hormones and great for the bowels)

A liberal amount of a high antioxidant juice like goji, pomegranate or acai (again, to pump up that immunity)

Quinoa Fit for a Queen

Quinoa is considered a grain, but is really the seed of the gooseberry plant. It is so amazing because, unlike any other "grain" out there, it is a complete protein. That means, Goddess, that eating a bowl of quinoa is like eating a piece of chicken or steak. It builds your muscles, revs your metabolism, and helps your brain. It has the added benefit of containing loads of B vitamins to help your energy, and lots of fibre to make your colon happy. You can use it as a porridge, in a salad, or just like you would rice. You have to rinse it first, as it is covered in saponin- a soapy like substance that helps the plant naturally ward of insects. Put it in a sieve and rinse until there are no more bubbles. Then cook it just like rice. Easy!

Ingredients:

1 cup quinoa, rinsed, and 2 cups water for cooking

1/2 cup goat feta, or more to taste

2 leaves kale, diced very fine, main stem removed (for calcium)

1 red pepper (for immune boosting vitamin C)

1 cucumber

1 clove garlic, minced (very anti viral)

1 can chickpeas, rinsed (more bone building calcium)

bunch of fresh basil or dill, chopped (anti viral, anti fungal)

Dressing:

1/2 cup best quality extra virgin olive oil or flax oil (or go half and half)

1/4 cup apple cider vinegar (Very alkalizing)

Sea salt and pepper to taste

Method:

After rinsing quinoa, cook it as you would rice. Place the 2 cups of water in a pot, add quinoa. Bring to boil, then turn down to a simmer. Allow it to cook, lid on, until water is absorbed. Quinoa is done when it is fluffy and the curly bits have separated from the round bits. Cool.

Chop all veggies, combine with quinoa. Add feta, chickpeas, herbs and dressing. Stir all together. Make a big batch and save some for lunches!

Heavenly Hummus

We need to keep our bones strong, Goddess. Hummus is full of calcium. Tahini (sesame paste) is extremely high in this bone building mineral, as are chickpeas. This recipe takes about 5 minutes in the food processor, and can be served with crudities or a nice whole grain pita or gluten free rice crackers.

Ingredients:

1 can rinsed chickpeas

3 tablespoons tahini

juice from 1/2 fresh lemon

2 cloves fresh garlic

sea salt to taste

water to blend.

Options:

- sprinkle in metabolism boosting spices such as cayenne or cumin for a kick
- roast a red pepper and toss it in for vitamin C
- add some feta for creaminess
- add 2 tablespoons flax oil for omega 3s and a smoother consistency.

Method:

Just toss it all in the food processor, and drizzle in the water until a creamy, paste-like consistency is reached.

Goddess Green Bowl

Sometimes goddesses have trouble figuring out how to use unusual dark green leafy vegetables in their daily lives. You see things like Swiss Chard and kale at the markets, but don't know how to make them taste good. It's really very simple. Both of these greens taste great raw or cooked. Their texture is a bit tough, so the best trick is to finely chop them and sprinkle them on whatever other vegetables you are eating. You can also lightly steam them. In this case, though, you would want to just wilt them enough to make them more chewable, a minute or so at most. Once you heat things past 118 degrees Fahrenheit, a lot of the vital nutrients are destroyed. The following recipe is quick and easy. You can even change up the ingredients to make it more kid or spouse friendly. The idea here though, is for you to be eating your veggies, so load up!

Ingredients:

3 leaves kale or Swiss Chard, centre vein stripped, leaves finely chopped

1 red pepper, sliced

1 zucchini, cubed

2 medium carrots, sliced into rounds

2 beets, grated

half red onion, sliced.

any other veggies of choice

1/2 cup broccoli crowns

fresh ginger to taste

1/4 cup hemp seeds

1/2 cup brown rice, cooked according to package directions

Dressing:

This is up to you. Adding a squeeze of lemon may be enough for you, or some chopped cilantro. If you like, you could add some Bragg's Seasoning (like soy sauce) or Tamari, tahini, and some garlic, ginger and honey to taste. Feel free to experiment with herbs and good for you flavors, they are nature's gift to your taste buds! Don't be afraid to make mistakes. This is the joy of food!

Method:

Chop veggies. Add a small amount of water to a skillet, and toss veggies in. Lightly steam veggies, starting with the harder ones like the broccoli. Add in the leaves at the very end. Only steam the veggies for 5 minutes or less.

Gorgeous Gourmet Coconut Almond Flatcakes

Goddess, sometimes it's nice to have a go-to recipe when you are feeling a little sweet. This batter recipe works amazingly well for both flatcakes and cookies. Do have fun, and enjoy divinely.

Ingredients:

1 cup spelt flour (50% less gluten than whole wheat)

1/2 cup almond flour (decadent, and contains calcium)

1/2 cup coconut (for hair, skin, eyes, and digestion)

1/4 cup oat bran (for gentle fibre)

1/4 cup flax meal, freshly ground (get those Omega 3s in ya!)

2 tsp aluminum free baking powder

pinch sea salt

1 egg (organic, free range)

2 more egg whites

1 teaspoon vanilla

1/4 cup unpasteurized honey (locally produced, if possible. One of nature's divine gifts. So good for you, there are books written on the subject.)

Milk or almond milk to moisten, if necessary

1 tbsp coconut oil (again, so amazing for you, and great for cooking at high heats.)

Dark chocolate chips, blueberries or raspberries to taste if desired.

Method 1:

Heat 1 tablespoon of coconut oil on skillet on medium low.

Combine all dry ingredients in bowl. Set aside.

Beat egg and egg whites together til fluffy. Add in honey, vanilla, and fold into dry ingredients.

Add in chocolate chips or blueberries, and use milk if necessary to get desired consistency. For pancakes, dough should be runny.

Pour batter in pan and flip when brown on one side. Serve with maple syrup, and sliced pears and pecans.

Method 2:

Preheat oven to 325 degrees fahrenheit.

Add less liquid and make cookie dough consistency.

Lay parchment paper on cookie sheet, spoon dough onto sheet, and bake for 8 minutes, or until golden.

Resources

Nourish

Blereau, Jude: *Wholefoods*

Davies, Barb and Rallison, Jennifer: *SLICE: Health Inspired Food Cookbook*

Eisenstein, Charles*: The Yoga of Eating*

Emoto, Masaru: *Messages From Water and many others*

Hobsbawn-Smith, dee: *Skinny Feasts; The Quick Gourmet; and The Curious Cook at Home*

Jensen, Dr. Bernard: *Dr. Jensen's Guide to Better Bowel Care: A Complete Program for Tissue Cleansing Through Bowel Management* ; *Empty Harvest; and more!*

Oliver, Jamie*: Jamie's Food Revolution and many others*

Pollan, Michael*: Food Rules, An Eater's Manual; The Omnivore's Dilemma; In Defense of Food*

Wolfe, David*: Naked Chocolate; Superfoods; and many others*

Uliano, Sophie*: Gorgeously Green*

Women's Health and Wellness

Hay, Louise: *You Can Heal Your Life*

Northrup, Dr. Christiane: *Women's Bodies, Women's Wisdom; The Wisdom of Menopause; The Power of Joy (audio recording)*

Williamson, Marianne: *A Woman's Worth; A Course In Miracles and many more!*

Acknowledgments

It isn't enough to just say thank you to all the lovely folks who have helped shape this book, let alone those who have helped shape our lives. But to all of you, the gratitude we feel for each of you is so immense, and so deep. We love you all and wish you buckets of joy.

To Gordon- Thank you for your years of subtle, profound teaching that has helped me find my way back to the surface, and on to solid ground. For your wisdom, I am eternally grateful. B.T.

To my daughters- May you grow as princesses, and blossom with grace and steadfast power into the unimaginable Goddesses you were born to be. I love you with all my heart. Thank you for being exactly who you are. Mom

To Mom, for all the little things you do for me that remind me that I am a Goddess, thank you. All my love. B.T.

To Dad, for quietly loving and supporting me, and for bringing humor to my life. I love you and miss you! B.T.

To my bro, for being such a great dude. There is still no one funnier than you. B.T.

To Chris, for your years of steadfast support and love that have gotten me from there to here. B.T.

To my Mother, Connie, my first teacher in the way of the Goddess. Thank you for showing me the value of women and the value of me. I love you, Mom.J.R.

To my children, each one of you is miraculous and awe inspiring to me and each day is a privilege to be apart of your lives. I dedicate this book to you because you all show me everyday that dreams really can come true. May you always know that yours can, too! Mom

To our own Goddess Gang. Thank you, girlfriends for being shoulders for crying, ears for listening, arms for hugging and souls for supporting. Whether we see each other every two days or two years makes no difference. You are the buttercream to our cake of life!!! xoxoxox

To all our trusted friends and advisors who have read, reread, edited, commented, and suggested improvements to make this book what it is, especially Sheila (mum to all), Meaghan, Stacey, Christene, Karen, Raphaelle and the gang at Icona . Thank you for your hard work and enthusiasm!!!

About the Goddesses

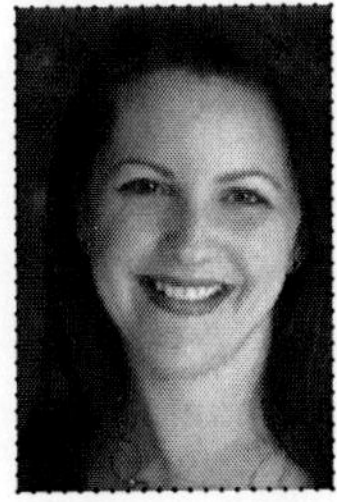

Barb Thomas, RHN

Barb is a Holistic Nutritionist/ Holistic Chef in private practice. When she is not shuttling her two mini-goddesses to their various lessons and social activities, she can be found teaching nutrition in Calgary, Alberta where she holds public and private whole foods cooking classes. Barb is a professional speaker and lectures frequently in the corporate sector. She can be reached at barb@love2eat.ca .

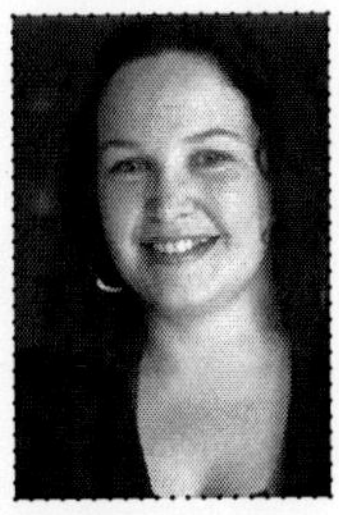

Jennifer Rochford

Mother of four very busy children who range in age from 3 all the way to 13, Jennifer spends her days in Edmonton, Alberta balancing motherhood with a full time career, a love for gourmet food, a lifelong passion for writing, and most recently, blogging professionally. Jenn can be reached, but only if you bribe her with french pastries.